UNDERSTANDING EVIDENCE-BASED PRACTICE

PRACTICE
FOR NURSING ASSOCIATES

UNDERSTANDING EVIDENCE-BASED PRACTICE

FOR NURSING ASSOCIATES

Melissa Owens
with
Jenny Adams, Peter Rogers
Hannah Smith & Vickie Welsh

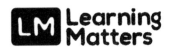

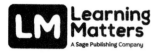

Learning Matters
A Sage Publishing Company
1 Oliver's Yard
55 City Road
London EC1Y 1SP

Sage Publications Inc.
2455 Teller Road
Thousand Oaks, California 91320

Sage Publications India Pvt Ltd
B 1/I 1 Mohan Cooperative Industrial Area
Mathura Road
New Delhi 110 044

Sage Publications Asia-Pacific Pte Ltd
3 Church Street
#10-04 Samsung Hub
Singapore 049483

Editor: Martha Cunneen
Development editor: Caroline Prodger
Senior project editor: Chris Marke
Marketing manager: Ruslana Khatagova
Cover design: Wendy Scott
Typeset by: C&M Digitals (P) Ltd, Chennai, India
Printed in the UK

Library of Congress number: 2024933059

British Library Cataloguing in Publication Data

A catalogue record for this book is available from the
British Library

ISBN 978-1-5296-0594-5
ISBN 978-1-5296-0593-8 (pbk)

Contents

About the authors   ix

Introduction   1

1   Providing evidence-based practice   5
     Vickie Welsh and Melissa Owens

2   Using evidence in contemporary practice   17
     Melissa Owens

3   Understanding research   31
     Melissa Owens

4   Critical appraisal of research   51
     Melissa Owens

5   Health inequalities, evidence-based practice and the nursing associate   71
     Hannah Smith

6   Decision-making in evidence-based practice: The law, ethics and values   83
     Jenny Adams

7   Change for quality improvement: Putting evidence into practice   99
     Peter Rogers

References   121
Index   131

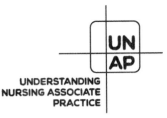

**UNDERSTANDING
NURSING ASSOCIATE
PRACTICE**

Supporting you through your nursing associate training & career

UNDERSTANDING NURSING ASSOCIATE PRACTICE is a series uniquely designed for trainee nursing associates.

Each book in the series is:
- Mapped to the NMC standards of proficiency for nursing associates
- Affordable
- Full of practical activities & case studies
- Focused on clearly explaining theory & its application to practice

Other books in the series include:

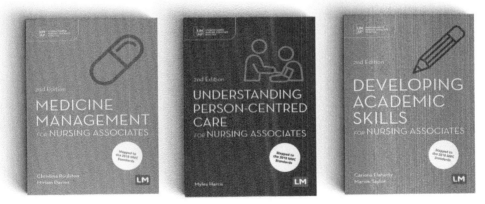

Visit
uk.sagepub.com/UNAP
to see the full collection

About the authors

Dr Melissa Owens (book editor) is Director of Nursing at the University of York and has responsibility for their Nursing and Nursing Associate Programmes. She has previously been a Nursing Associate Programme Leader. She has a particular interest in evidence-based practice, which forms a major part of her teaching. She is a Registered Nurse: Learning Disabilities and her research and publications have an educational focus. Melissa also has a particular interest in interprofessional education and is a Board member of CAIPE (Centre for the Advancement of Interprofessional Education) and co-leads their Faculty Develop Sub-Group. She previously led their Research Development Sub-Group and in November 2023 was part of a team who won an International Global Award for interprofessional team working. She completed her Doctorate of Education in 2015, which focused on collaborative working in primary care.

Jenny Adams is an Assistant Professor at the University of Bradford and developed the original pilot Foundation Degree (Science) Nursing Associate Programme as well as the current NMC approved programme. She continues to act as module leader for two of the level 4 modules on the programme. In addition, she has developed undergraduate and postgraduate programmes in non-medical prescribing and advanced practice. Her clinical experience was mostly as a health visitor and practice development nurse in the community setting. Jenny is an enthusiastic teacher and passionate about developing safe nursing practice to meet the changing demands of healthcare.

Peter Rogers is an Assistant Professor at the University of Bradford and has been involved in the delivery of the Foundation Degree (Science) Nursing Associate Programme at the University of Bradford since its inception in 2017. Peter acted as deputy programme leader for the original pilot of the programme and continues to be actively involved in its delivery. Prior to joining the University of Bradford Peter held positions within both NHS England and the NHS Clinical Governance Support Team, where as Associate Director of Education he was responsible for developing and leading clinical service improvement programmes across the NHS in England and supporting similar developments in Wales and Northern Ireland. After the dissolution of the NHS Modernisation Agency, he held a number of consultancy positions supporting change projects ranging from national programmes, including CfH and the NHS Integrated Service Improvement Programme, to others designed to deliver service improvements at NHS Trust level. Peter is module leader for the final level 5 module which focuses on improving care quality, including a significant level of content relating to evidence-based practice.

Hannah Smith is a freelance nurse and lecturer who worked as a Lecturer at the University of Bradford for two years, during which time she was the deputy programme lead for the Foundation Degree (Science) Nursing Associate Programme, and was also involved in the delivery. Hannah was the module leader for their first level 5 module which focuses on integrated care. She also taught on postgraduate critical care modules, and has a particular interest in promoting equity and inclusivity. Prior to commencing at the university, Hannah worked as a clinical nurse educator in critical care and has almost 20 years of acute care experience, both as a nurse and midwife.

Vickie Welsh is a Senior Lecturer at the University of Leeds and leads the Independent and Supplementary Prescribing module for Nurses and Midwives. She was involved in the delivery of the Foundation Degree (Science) Nursing Associate Programme at the University of Bradford, where she offered specific support to small employers in the practice setting and assisted in the development and delivery of clinical skills. Vickie is enthusiastic about supporting students both in university and in clinical practice to ensure they meet their goals and succeed.

Introduction

Who is this book for?

Thank you for choosing to read our book on understanding evidence-based practice for nursing associates. This book has been written with those learning to be a nursing associate in mind. However, it is equally relevant for any student and healthcare professional who needs an easy-to-follow text to help improve their understanding of the underlying principles of evidence-based practice and support to develop the skills to deliver it.

About the book

Our book focuses on evidence-based practice for nursing associates. Evidence-based practice is a core capability that is a requirement of the Nursing and Midwifery Council (NMC)'s *Standards of Proficiency for Nursing Associates*. The NMC defines evidence-based person-centred care as 'making sure that any care and treatment is given to people by looking at what research has shown to be most effective' (NMC, 2018b).

   This book sets out to equip you to learn, develop and embed this essential skill with confidence. The focus of our book is a practical one and aims to equip you with both the knowledge and skills to enhance your practice and ensure it is evidence-based. The book is loosely divided into two halves with the first half offering a more practical focus on developing your skills and the second half focusing on widening and deepening your knowledge.

Book structure

Our book is made up of seven chapters, each looking at evidence-based practice with a different focus. After this introduction, the book will guide you through the essential skills you will need to ensure your own practice is evidence-based. We provide a step-by-step guide to database searching, before introducing you to the basic principles of research and how to critique it. We then move on to help you consider how evidence-based practice is delivered when applied to different patient groups, and the ethical dilemmas you are likely to face in your practice. Finally, we get you to think about the concept of change. Providing 'better', evidence-based healthcare can mean having to change practice. Therefore, this concluding chapter helps you to consider how you can contribute to the process of change in a systematic way, in order to improve the evidence-based care you provide.

   Chapter 1 introduces the concept of evidence-based practice and takes you on a journey through the history of how it developed. We include some real-life examples from a nurse called 'Margaret' who tells us about her experience of nursing in the 1950s. We explore what was important in nursing care then, in comparison to contemporary practice, today: of ritualistic practices in comparison to evidence-based ones. While ritualistic practices do still occur today, we get you to reflect on your own practice and consider why you do something in the way you do and the evidence-base behind it.

Chapter 2 asks you to consider different types of evidence and why some are more reliable sources than others. We take you, step-by-step, through the principles and practicalities of undertaking a database search to find evidence to support and improve your practice and introduce you to a case study of the real-life experiences of 'Simon'. We then use this case study as a working example to help you develop skills to find 'good' evidence to support his care in a systematic way.

Chapter 3 introduces you to the principles of research: of the differences between quantitative and qualitative research, the principles, terminologies and methods used in each. Our experience suggests many trainee nursing associates are daunted by the prospect of reading research articles, so our core aim in this chapter is to demystify the terminology used in research and to boost your confidence by making research less intimidating and more accessible. To help you we introduce you to another case study: an adolescent called Toni who identifies as transgender; by applying what we have learnt we show you how research can be used to help you decide how to best meet the care needs of Toni.

Chapter 4 builds on Chapter 3 by taking you through the principles and skills of critiquing research. We start by helping you to think about how you already use critical skills in everyday practice, as well as outlining why it is important to critique research to ensure it is credible, robust and relevant. We introduce tools to help you critique research systematically and return to the case study of Toni to explore how different research can, and cannot, help you better care for your patients.

Chapter 5 focuses on health inequalities and how important it is to consider the needs of all those you care for in an inclusive and culturally competent way. We explore why 'good' health is not enjoyed by all and the social determinants that can impact on both individual health and length of life. We consider how protected characteristics, as outlined in the Equality Act (2010), can intersect with health inequalities, and encourage you to reflect on the care that you provide in this context. In addition, we look at how standardised care can overlook some patient groups, meaning they are likely to have poorer outcomes than others.

Chapter 6 explores how ethical decision-making can be used as a tool for evidence-based practice. In addition to research, understanding and applying the principles of ethical and legal frameworks is essential for nursing associates. We use the case example of Jim, an older adult with reduced capacity to make decisions and consent, to help you explore the balancing act of weighing up evidence-based care with ethical and legal considerations.

Chapter 7 is the closing chapter of the book and here we introduce you to the theory underpinning service improvement. Ensuring practice is evidence-based often requires practices to change in order to improve and, in this final chapter, we introduce you to service improvement theories, to help you consider how change can be introduced into your practice in a structured way. We introduce you to three service improvement models and include a number of activities, including a case study, to help you work through the systematic process of introducing evidence-based change.

Requirements for the NMC *Standards of Proficiency for Nursing Associates*

The NMC has established standards of proficiency to be met by applicants to different parts of the register, and these are the standards it considers necessary for safe and effective practice.

This book is structured so that it will help you to understand and meet the proficiencies required for entry to the NMC register as a nursing associate. The relevant proficiencies are presented at the start of each chapter so that you can clearly see which ones the chapter addresses. The proficiencies have been designed to be generic so apply to all fields of nursing and all care settings. This is because nursing associates must be able to meet the needs of any person they encounter in their practice regardless of their stage of life or health challenges, whether these are mental, physical, cognitive or behavioural. We, therefore, introduce a number of different case studies and learning activities across the chapters within our book to reflect this and help you apply the knowledge and skills you gain to different health settings and patient groups.

This book includes the latest standards for 2018 onwards, taken from the *Standards of Proficiency for Nursing Associates* (NMC, 2018a).

Learning features

Textbooks can be intimidating and learning from reading text is not always easy. However, this series has been designed specifically to help the nursing associate learn from the books within it. The various learning features throughout the books will help you to develop your understanding and ability to apply theory to practice, while remaining engaging and breaking the text up into manageable chunks. This book contains activities, case studies, theory summary boxes, further reading, useful websites and other materials to enable you to participate in your own learning. The book cannot provide all the answers – but instead provides a good outline of the most important information and helps you build a framework for your own learning.

As we highlight above, as a nursing associate you will work across a variety of settings and different patient groups. With this in mind, we provide you with a number of learning activities that reflect this. This includes a series of different case scenarios.

Answers to all the activities in the book are provided. It is important to attempt the activities and to read the answers thoroughly against your own responses, to ensure you have fully understood the concepts explored. This will help you obtain the maximum value from the activities by reinforcing your learning.

We include a number of additional learning features to support you to develop your learning in relation to all the topics we cover in our book and hope you find them useful and an enjoyable way of learning. Good luck with your studies!

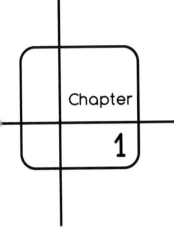

Chapter

1

Providing evidence-based practice

Vickie Welsh and Melissa Owens

NMC STANDARDS OF PROFICIENCY FOR NURSING ASSOCIATES

This chapter will address the following platforms and proficiencies:

Platform 1: Being an accountable professional

1.1 understand and act in accordance with the Code: Professional standards of practice and behaviour for nurses, midwives, nursing associates, and fulfil all registration requirements

1.17 safely demonstrate evidence based practice in all skills and procedures stated in Annexes A and B

Platform 4: Working in teams

4.9 discuss the influence of policy and political drivers that impact health and care provision

Chapter aims

After reading this chapter you will be able to:

- understand the meaning of evidence-based practice and how it relates to your role as a nursing associate;
- recognise how care has changed over time due to an evidence-based understanding of care practices;
- develop an awareness that evidence-based practice is fundamental to the NMC's Standards.

Introduction

As a nursing associate, you will be caring for a variety of patients in different settings and with varying needs. You are required to put the interests of your patients first and ensure that the care and treatments you provide are evidence-based. You will do this by working in accordance with the Standards identified within the NMC Code (NMC, 2018a) which is broken down into four sections as shown in Figure 1.1:

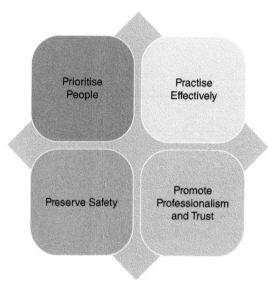

Figure 1.1 The four standards of the NMC Code (2018a)

Upon registration as a nursing associate you will be required to commit to working professionally, safely and effectively and to uphold the Standards of the Code (NMC, 2018a).

Evidence-based practice is a fundamental element of each of these standards and in this chapter we will begin by examining what is meant by the term 'evidence-based practice'. We will also explore the journey that nursing has taken towards becoming evidence-based in its delivery, and its relevance to you as a nursing associate. Using critical thinking activities, we will determine why the use of evidence-based healthcare is important and why this should be chosen as a priority over traditions, routines and rituals in helping you to achieve the Standards within the Code (NMC, 2018a).

Many nursing associates have previous experience as healthcare support workers (HCSW). As you progress into becoming a nursing associate, however, the expectations increase, and you become accountable to the NMC. As a HCSW you know what to do and how to do it but as a nursing associate there is a requirement that you also understand *why* you are doing what you are doing. As you read above, the NMC Code (2018a) requires you to practise effectively and to ensure that any care or treatments you give are evidence-based. Similarly, the NMC *Standards of Proficiency for Nursing Associates* (2018b) stipulate that when making care/treatment decisions you should look at what research has shown to be most effective while considering your own judgement and experience alongside the views and preferences of the person receiving the treatment – that is, that you are providing evidence-based practice. It is therefore essential that you fully understand what evidence-based practice is and how to apply it to those within your care.

As a healthcare professional you cannot assume that any nursing procedure demonstrated to you is evidence-based. We have to consider why you might not observe evidence-based practice.

Usually, the decision *not* to utilise evidence-based practice is unlikely to be a deliberate choice made by the demonstrator. It might be that a policy has recently changed, or that new evidence has also recently come to light. However, it might be that the demonstrator is carrying out that procedure without thinking about the evidence behind it because they have always done it that way. As we will discuss within this chapter, there were many practices based on tradition. Some of these might remain today and you could, unconsciously, be practising these.

What does evidence-based practice mean?

You may have heard the term before, but it is important to understand what evidence-based practice actually means. Let's look at a definition:

> **Evidence-based practice** is the integration of the *best research evidence* with *patient values* and *clinical expertise*, while considering the resources available (Dawes et al., 2005).

All three elements – best research evidence, patient values and clinical expertise – hold equal importance. Evidence-based practice within nursing, in particular, is the idea that all nursing practice should be based on scientific information while also considering what the patient wants and the expertise of the healthcare professionals. Basing our practice on evidence requires us to take an active approach to providing care in a non-biased, individualistic way. Using evidence-based practice also results in a more consistent approach across health services (Thompson et al., 2004).

It is important to note that in terms of research evidence, the 'best available' may be different for each situation. Not only is new information being generated all the time, but also, conclusive evidence may not always exist for every question or problem, particularly for those who have multiple comorbidities or conditions. To add to the complications, just because a treatment is shown to be the most effective does not mean it will be recommended in local or national policy; many considerations are taken into account when healthcare policy and guidelines are created.

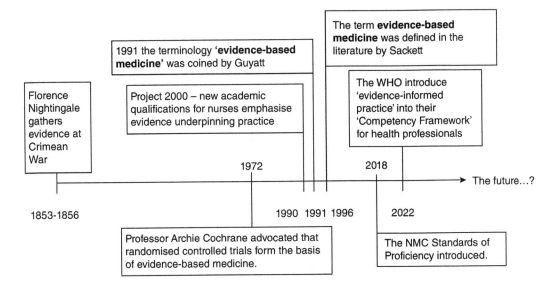

Figure 1.2 A timeline showing the evolution of evidence-based practice

For example, there may be a drug which is 80 per cent effective at treating a condition, but this drug might cost several hundred thousand pounds per dose. There is a second drug which is also 80 per cent effective, but costs just a few pounds per dose, although will incur more side effects for the receiving patient. Policy may choose to advocate for the second drug in this situation, despite knowing that the first is better for the patient. Even so, it is important to remain aware of best practice.

Historical development of evidence-based practice

So, how did evidence-based practice evolve? In the next section we look at the timeline shown in Figure 1.2.

The 1850s: Florence Nightingale

In the era of Florence Nightingale, the term 'evidence-based practice' had not yet been invented. However, if we look at her work, it is clear to see that evidence-based practice was fundamental in the nursing care she endeavoured to provide to her patients. After the Crimean war (1853–6), Nightingale was intent that such a loss of life would not happen again. She understood that data and statistics were essential for improvement. She was the first to gather and utilise statistics to enhance the understanding and evaluation of progress to improve patient outcomes. In observing and understanding the information she collected she found that British soldiers were less likely to die as a result of their injuries and more likely to die as a result of disease contracted from unsanitary conditions. When Nightingale conducted a study of maternal mortality from puerperal fever, she found that maternal mortality rates were much higher for those who were inpatients than those who were cared for at home. Based on the evidence she had collated, Nightingale closed the midwifery ward and associated training school (Lloyd, 2020), one of the first clear evidence-based decisions.

The 1970s: Professor Archie Cochrane

Fast forward to the 1970s and evidence-based practice was beginning to find its place in the medical profession. In 1972, Professor Archie Cochrane, a doctor, expressed concerns that treatment decisions were rarely based on clinical evidence. An international collaboration followed which highlighted the gap between clinical practice and research and started to convince practitioners of the value of evidence-based practice. Cochrane indicated that only procedures which had been proven to be effective should be utilised, mostly due to a predicted limitation in resources. Cochrane advocated that randomised controlled trials should form the foundation of clinical decision-making and this evolved into the evidence-based medicine movement.

The 1990s: Gordon Guyatt, Sackett and Project 2000

In 1991 the terminology 'evidence-based medicine' was coined by Gordon Guyatt and his team (the Evidence-based Medicine Working Group), who attempted to shift the focus on clinical decision-making to be based on scientific research evidence rather than unsystematic clinical experience. The term was first mentioned in a small editorial wherein Guyatt attempted to explain the application of evidence-based medicine (Guyatt, 1991). The team, however, first published in the medical literature in 1992 and introduced the concept of evidence-based practice as something which would improve patient care by relying more on factual evidence and less on subjective clinician opinion (Guyatt et al., 1992).

Despite the prior publications by Guyatt, a clear definition of the term 'evidence-based medicine' was not clearly identified until 1996 when David Sackett described it as: 'the conscientious, explicit and judicious use of current best evidence in making decisions about the care of individual patients' (Sackett et al., 1996: 71). Sackett et al. went on to recommend that evidence, research and patient preference and beliefs should all be taken into account in order to fully utilise evidence-based medicine.

Within nursing, evidence-based healthcare began to take shape with the introduction of the Project 2000 scheme, which was rolled out across the country from 1990. Under this scheme, pre-registration nurse education moved from an apprenticeship-type model, taking place in individual hospitals, to higher education establishments/colleges. The final award had academic standing: initially at diploma level (what we now call a foundation degree) before moving to the degree (and sometimes masters level) qualification that we know today. Students undertook an 18-month common foundation programme, followed by 18 months specialising in their chosen branch (now field). Students no longer formed part of the workforce but were supernumerary, meaning they were in addition to the usual number of staff, and the importance of evidence underpinning practice was emphasised. For the first time, students were encouraged to question and think independently, rather than simply 'doing' as students had previously done (Parker and Carlisle, 1996). The curriculum changed meaning student nurses learnt about conducting and utilising research in clinical practice. However, a review of the literature found that following Project 2000 there was only a 10 per cent increase in nurses reporting they used research in practice (Parahoo, 1999) highlighting this was just the start of the changes required to nurse education programmes to embed evidence-based practice.

The present day

Trainee nursing associate programmes, we could argue, mirror some of what the 'old' nursing programmes looked like in that they are, predominantly, apprenticeship-based and are salaried. However, the similarity ends there as the affiliation with higher education establishments/colleges means that the final award has academic standing and, as such, requires you also to be a questioning, independent thinker who underpins your practice with evidence (NMC, 2018b). One of the criticisms of Project 2000 was that students didn't feel sufficiently prepared for practice because not enough emphasis was placed on the acquisition of clinical skills (Parker and Carlise, 1996). Consequently, pre-registration programmes today emphasise the attainment of skills by the point of registration through the NMC Standards of Proficiencies. These are known as the *Future Nurse: Standards of Proficiency for Registered Nurses* (NMC, 2018c) and the NMC *Standards of Proficiency for Nursing Associates* (NMC, 2018b). Although the Standards were introduced in 2018, the model continues to be considered best practice. Indeed, WHO since published a *Competency Framework* which identifies key competencies (domains) that should be included in the educational programmes of all healthcare professionals worldwide, including a domain they call 'evidence-informed practice' (what we refer to in this book as 'evidence-based practice') (WHO, 2022).

Have a read of this real-life case study, written by a retired nurse who started her nursing career as a student nurse in the 1950s.

Case study: Margaret

Margaret was asked: what was it like to be a student nurse in the 1950s? Here is part of what Margaret said:

(Continued)

(Continued)

'The first thing we were taught was how to dress. We had to wear an ironed dress, black tights and laced-up shoes with a lacey cap on our heads, with white grips. We had long sleeves with frilly cuffs that were removable, and a large, metal belt. We had to dress smartly as it showed that we were important and knew what we were doing. We would have to remove our cuffs and roll up our sleeves to care for a patient but if matron came in, we had to quickly roll our sleeves back down and try to put our cuffs back on, behind our back. If matron ever caught us with our sleeves rolled up, we would be in trouble.'

Source: Narrated by a retired nurse and used here with permission.

Activity 1.1   Critical thinking

The way that you dress now as a nursing associate will be very different to the way that Margaret was expected to dress as a student nurse in the 1950s. When Margaret was a student nurse, presentation and appearance were of paramount importance (Houweling, 2004). Consider how you are expected to dress today and the reasons behind it. Read the description Margaret provided of her uniform and consider what evidence might have been found that resulted in a change of uniform.

An outline answer is provided at the end of this chapter.

Our understanding of evidence-based healthcare is now far greater than in the 1950s and we also consider issues from a variety of different perspectives. Although public (and patient) confidence remains important, so too does comfort, the practicalities of doing your job and infection control: the latter has become even more important since the start of the COVID-19 pandemic (Shbaklo et al., 2021). The nursing cap that Margaret wore, for example, was abolished in the 1980s, not only because it was considered impractical and got in the way when carrying out intimate care, but it was also found to harbour germs and was difficult to clean (Dolan, 1983; Halliwell and Nayda, 2011).

We also started to become more aware of sex discrimination and differences in the 1960s and 70s (Houweling, 2004): male nurses at the time did not have to wear a cap for example, so why should female nurses have to? While professional appearance is still considered important, comfort and practicalities now take precedence over presentation (Spragley and Francis, 2006) with nurses, like many other healthcare professionals, commonly now wearing scrubs (Bates, 2023). Consider, for example, trying to undertake a moving and handling procedure which requires you to kneel on the bed, if you were wearing a dress.

Case study: Margaret (continued)

Many other things have changed too. For example, have a look at this additional comment that Margaret made regarding being a student nurse in the 1950s:

'When you arrived on the ward at the start of your shift, the staff nurse would go into sister's office to take the handover and we hung around outside waiting.'

Source: Narrated by a retired nurse and used here with permission.

Activity 1.2 Critical thinking

There are a variety of different ways that handovers are carried out today, but generally you will always be included in the handover as a nursing associate. Can you identify different ways in which handovers are now carried out? What is the evidence-base behind them?

An outline answer is provided at the end of this chapter.

You may not have previously considered patient handover in relation to evidence-based practice, but there is now a recognised association between good handovers and patient safety. Specifically, communication problems during handover have been identified as the cause of errors being made in patient care. Consequently, it is important that you learn handover and communication skills early in your career (Kim et al., 2021). An important aim of the handover is to transfer the responsibility and accountability of care from one set of professionals to another, requiring all relevant information to be communicated effectively (Pun, 2021). However, patient values are also an important part of evidence-based healthcare and, therefore, you might have included bedside handover in your list of different types of handovers in the activity above. This type of handover not only helps improve patient safety through including the patient's perspective, but it also improves patient and family satisfaction (Jimmerson et al., 2021). Handovers don't just take place in the acute hospital setting either. They are just as important in the community where one team is handing over care, or treatment, of complex patients to another team (Gray, 2020). Handovers also tend to be more structured than they were when Margaret was a student. Using a tool, such as SBAR (situation, background, assessment and recommendation), for example, is not uncommon to ensure all the key points that need to be communicated are included (Park, 2020).

Traditions, routines and rituals

As we highlighted earlier in this chapter, Project 2000 was arguably a key turning point in terms of pre-registration nursing and the focus on evidence-based healthcare. Prior to this, and certainly in the years when Margaret was a student nurse, there was a much greater emphasis on traditions, routines, rituals and taken-for-granted practices that tended to be task-focused and to continue because 'they have always been done that way'. Students weren't encouraged to think, and certainly not to challenge, but to do as they were told without questioning (Laurent, 2019).

Even though the nursing associate is still a relatively new profession, you continue to work alongside established professions and it can be easy to slip into the habits of a task-oriented way of working without even realising that it has happened (Nairn et al., 2012). A task-oriented approach is concerned with making the life of the nurse (and the nursing associate) easier, rather than benefitting the patient. This can be particularly true if you have previously worked as a HCSW.

Activity 1.3 Reflection

Have you ever worked (or know of) anywhere which has 12-hour shifts in place? These continue to be common today and yet there is now lots of evidence to show that it can impact negatively on both patients and staff. Despite how long we've known this, they continue to this day. Why do you think this is?

An outline answer is provided at the end of this chapter.

If you have worked 12-hour shifts it may be that you hadn't previously questioned whether they were good or not for practice. However, questioning what you see is an important part of ensuring evidence-based practice.

Working alongside others, but not questioning practices, can also have serious consequences on the safety of our patients. The Francis Inquiry (2013), for example, was carried out after it was identified that up to 1200 patients had died within a period of 50 months as a direct result of poor care at Mid Staffordshire NHS Trust, alongside significant suffering of others. The aim of the Inquiry was to examine the cause of these failings. Some examples of the failings that the Inquiry highlighted were as a result of tolerance of poor standards of care across many different professions and agencies. Sadly, this is not a unique example and as such the NMC (as well as all other professional and regulatory bodies) recognise the importance of your working collaboratively and include this in your Standards of Proficiency (NMC, 2018b).

Nevertheless, traditions and routines continue to be passed on. If you are immersed in routines and task-focused, taken-for-granted care practices, how do you know that the care you and others are providing is evidence-based? It is important that you understand why you are doing what you are doing. As a trainee it is easy to fall into the trap of following what qualified staff might do, or tell you to do, and what you see others doing in practice. However, it is your responsibility to ensure that you provide the most up-to-date and evidence-based practice you could be using, and to question and challenge others when you see something that appears to be based on tradition, rather than evidence-based.

Below is a selection of real-life examples of care that was based on tradition or routine rather than evidence. While some are now quite dated, other examples are more recent.

Case study: Examples of care

'When I practised as a mental health nurse in the 1960s and 70s, it was commonplace to confiscate personal clothing and hand out standard-issue clothing every morning. This would then be collected in during the evening and nightgowns handed out. There was little consideration in regards to the fit of an item of clothing, or the personal identity of the wearer.'

'On my very first shift as a student nurse for people with a learning disability, in 1983, I was given a kidney bowl and a set of nail clippers and told to remove the tights of the 30 elderly women on the ward and to cut their toenails – irrespective of whether they all needed them cutting or not.'

'In the 1980s you were allowed to smoke in the day rooms on the wards in general hospitals. In 1985 I was admitted to hospital with an acute appendicitis and got talking to the older woman in the bed opposite who was admitted to have her diet reviewed, prior to a surgical procedure. This one lunchtime the older woman asked the nurse if she could eat by her bed, rather than go to the day room, as it smelt of cigarette smoke in there and put her off her food. The nurse refused this request and told her she either had to go to the day room or go without her lunch. The woman decided on the latter.'

'As a nursing student, in the noughties, I was astounded when on placement on an elderly ward to find that it was expected that staff would wake up patients from 4am onwards to start their morning routine in order to make the day shift "easier". Attitudes such as this can be difficult to alter.'

'In 2018 my frail, elderly, stepfather could no longer get himself out of bed. Consequently, he was reliant on two carers coming to the house to hoist him into bed at night and out again in the morning. However, due to the shifts the carers worked he would often be in bed by 8 o'clock each night and not got up again until 10 o'clock the following morning.'

'In 2023 I was in the Emergency Department with my frail, elderly, mother-in-law. She'd slipped down the bed and the junior doctor asked me to help lift her back up it again. I was aware of the evidence-base behind *not* using bed sheets to slide patients and told her I would help if she found a slide sheet. She went away and returned with the charge nurse and between them proceeded to use the bed sheet to slide my mother-in-law back up the bed.'

Source: Narrated by colleagues and used here with their permission.

Activity 1.4   Critical thinking and reflection

Think about the care you provide on a day-to-day basis. Do any of these examples resonate? Consider how you know the care you provide is evidence-based and not simply based on tradition or routine or, if it is, how you could do it differently.

As this answer is based on your own observation, there is no outline answer at the end of the chapter.

While some of these examples may now sound out-dated, time constraints and lack of equipment, as well as a keenness to conform and fit in with the team, can sometimes lead to a tendency to default to routine-based practices (Nairn et al., 2012). Equally, healthcare provision only has finite resources and although the NHS is a not-for-profit organisation it still has financial constraints which will impact the number of professionals and healthcare workers that are available in any given area (Bradshaw and Bradshaw, 2004). The ageing of our population means that the frail, elderly gentleman in the example above was one of a number of older adults who needed help getting into and out of bed from a finite number of healthcare workers. The next time you observe or take part in a nursing procedure, ask yourself if you know why it is being done that way. If you don't know, ask the person you are observing to see if they can tell you. Hopefully they will be able to give you an answer, but, if not, you can find out how to find the evidence later in this book.

Chapter summary

This first chapter provides a foundation to your understanding of evidence-based practice and why it is important. The examples of traditional practices we provide help emphasise how healthcare practices can be delivered in a task-focused, rather than patient-focused, way. However, taken-for-granted traditions of working still occur today and it is all too easy to slip into routines of others without questioning. Consequently, it can impact not only the quality of care, but also the safety of care provided. As we saw from the Mid Staffordshire NHS Trust example (Francis, 2013) above, patients do die when care is poor and unquestioned. This can be particularly true if you were previously a HCSW and learnt to carry out your tasks without considering the evidence behind the care you were giving. As a nursing associate it is important that you learn to question and challenge both your own practices and those of others in order to avoid slipping into taken-for-granted ways of working. In the next chapter, and beyond, we will help you to develop your skills further in order to learn how to find evidence-based literature (Chapter 2), understand the principles of research (Chapter 3) and then ascertain the quality of it (Chapter 4) before considering, in subsequent chapters, how and where you might apply it.

Activities: Brief outline answers

Activity 1.1 Critical thinking

When Margaret was a student nurse the primary aim of a uniform appeared to be appearance, in order to instil respect from those they nursed. Although public confidence is still recognised as important in the wearing of uniforms (Desta et al., 2015), it is only one of a number of things that are now considered. Infection control, for example, now recognises long sleeves, and indeed cuffs of any sort, to be inappropriate as they can become heavily contaminated and therefore should not be worn (RCN, 2017a). Moving and handling techniques now recognise that the nurse's buckle can injure a patient. The comfort of staff is also recognised to be important and there is now even consideration of the type of fibre used in a uniform to ensure women who are menopausal, or peri-menopausal, can remain comfortable (NHS, 2020). In addition, the practicality of the uniform is important. Few females now wear dresses as there is also a requirement that uniforms should fit well and enable easy movement (HSE, 1992).

Activity 1.2 Critical thinking

Patient handover has changed dramatically over the years as recognition of its importance in relation to patient safety has grown (Kim et al., 2021). Unlike when Margaret was a student in the 1950s, it's now normal for all staff to be involved in the handover to ensure they are fully aware of the needs of the patients they will be responsible for while on duty, in order to ensure patient safety.

There are now also different types of handovers that are used. Bedside handover, for example, is one and is now considered the 'gold standard' handover as it not only helps enhance patient safety, but it is also considered to enhance patient and family satisfaction, as they are active participants in the process (Jimmerson et al., 2021).

You may also have identified a 'huddle'. Although slightly different from the traditional handover, its goals are still to ensure patient safety and still include many elements of the traditional handover. One important element is that a huddle includes members of the multidisciplinary team (MDT) rather than just nursing staff in order to achieve common goals (Gray, 2020; McBeth, 2017).

There are a number of tools that can be used to bring structure to the handover and ensure all relevant information is included. SBAR, for example, can be used as a checklist to ensure not only that the key information is relayed, but also that irrelevant details are not included (Park, 2020).

Activity 1.3 Reflection

There are many reasons 12-hour shifts continue to be commonplace. You might have thought of answers such as flexibility. The National Nursing Research Unit (Ball et al., 2014) found that some nurses reported they preferred them due to greater flexibility and better work–life balance. Some nurses also felt they were better off financially as they could pick up extra shifts on their non-working days.

Annotated further reading

Aveyard, H and Sharp, P (2017) *A Beginner's Guide to Evidence-Based Practice in Health and Social Care* (3rd edition). London: McGraw-Hill Education.

This book is a great place to start. It uses easy-to-understand language to help describe what evidence-based practice is, how to relate it to practice and how to use it within your academic work.

Francis, R (2013) *Report of the Mid Staffordshire NHS Foundation Trust Public Inquiry.* February. London: HMSO. Available at: https://assets.publishing.service.gov.uk/government/uploads/system/uploads/attachment_data/file/279124/0947.pdf

This is the full report into the Inquiry discussed in this chapter.

Laurent, C (2019) *Rituals and Myths in Nursing: A Social History.* Barnsley: Pen and Sword History.

This text describes a number of personal experiences of nurses, capturing the developments of an evidence-based approach in nurse training.

Useful websites

www.rmmonline.co.uk

The Royal Marsden Manual of Clinical Procedures online provides step-by-step guides for each clinical skill, with rationale provided for each step. In addition, the manual critically discusses the evidence-base which encompasses a wide variety of sources, including patient feedback.

https://bestpractice.bmj.com/info/toolkit

This website provides an introduction to evidence-based practice with a further reading list.

https://bestpractice.bmj.com

In partnership with Higher Education England, the British Medical Journal provides an award-winning resource for healthcare professionals. This digital tool provides easily accessible evidence-based research, guidelines and expert opinion which is updated daily.

https://guides.mclibrary.duke.edu/ebptutorial

A tutorial introducing you to the principles of evidence-based healthcare.

https://s4be.cochrane.org/

A network for students interested in evidence-based healthcare.

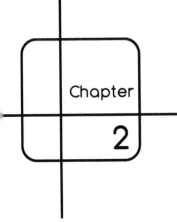

Chapter

2

Using evidence in contemporary practice

Melissa Owens

NMC STANDARDS OF PROFICIENCY FOR NURSING ASSOCIATE

This chapter will address the following platforms and proficiencies:

Platform 1: Being an accountable professional

1.1   understand and act in accordance with the Code: Professional standards of practice and behaviour for nurses, midwives and nursing associates, and fulfil all registration requirements

1.16   act as an ambassador for their profession and promote public confidence in health and care services

1.17   safely demonstrate evidence based practice in all skills and procedures in Annexes A and B

Chapter aims

After reading this chapter you will be able to:

- appreciate what makes good evidence for use in practice;
- recognise the place of evidence in ensuring effective patient care;
- create a list of search terms using a PICO(S) and PCC search tool;
- demonstrate understanding of how to carry out a database search using a recognised database searching tool.

Introduction

Nursing associates are registered healthcare professionals and as such must abide by the Nursing and Midwifery (NMC) Code (2018a). As we discussed in Chapter 1, the Code is made up of four elements. The second of these is 'Practise effectively' and requires you to ensure that everything you do is evidence-based. This means you can't simply follow what someone else tells you to do. Instead, you must play an active role in discussing the care you give with others and ensuring you base your own care on what the research suggests is the best evidence available (NMC, 2018a, b). In this chapter we explore this concept further and help you develop the tools you need to be able to achieve this. Reading this chapter will take you through the different types of evidence that can be used to support your practice and through the process of carrying out a database search step by step. We use a short case study to help illustrate the examples used in this chapter but also encourage you to reflect on the how and where you might use the skills you learn within your everyday practice.

Read the following case study of an individual living with a long-term health condition. Simon (aged 32) tells the story of his life living with an ileostomy and the health challenges he faces.

Case study: Simon

Simon was asked: 'How do you experience life, living with a long-term health condition?' Here is Simon's story.

'Having a stoma takes over every aspect of your life. As it contributes to a bodily function that you no longer have control over, you need to prepare for how this will affect you, both mentally and physically.

I had a sub-total colectomy, to remove part of my bowel, when I was just 26. I had been suffering from an ulcerative colitis flare-up that couldn't be controlled medically and had been in constant pain for nine months before my surgery.

Before leaving hospital, I was talked through the practicalities of living with a stoma: how to empty and clean my bag; how to change it when required and where to order further supplies. Initially, coping with an ileostomy bag was daunting, but, thankfully, my now wife helped me through the early days. For example, not long after returning home she ended up having to clean me up after my bag had overfilled as I couldn't bend forward.

Following my surgery, I had to totally change my diet and consider what and when I ate. Some foods, for example, could block the stoma. I learnt the hard way that a chickpea curry was something that I couldn't eat while my body was still adjusting to the stoma. I was also advised to eat little and often (something I struggle with to this day) as a large meal could fill (or overfill) my ileostomy bag with little or no warning. Alcohol affects me more now too, meaning I can only tolerate small amounts in comparison to what I could drink before.

I've continued to have health problems since the surgery and had to take steroids for a long time. I suffer from vitamin D deficiency and must take supplements every day. The fatigue and leg pain I feel are definitely not pleasant and earlier this year I fractured my shoulder socket with no explanation. Although I can't be sure this was exacerbated by my vitamin D deficiency, I suspect that it was.

Having a sub-total colectomy meant that they left some of my colon intact, but I have continued to have flare-ups of ulcerative colitis and on occasions these have lasted for several months. I work in the emergency services and this has affected my ability to work during these times. I am now on the waiting list for a total proctocolectomy. I don't yet fully know how this will impact my life but whatever it brings, I am hopeful that it will be positive.'

Source: This case study was provided by the service user with permission to use it in this publication.

Activity 2.1　Critical thinking and reflection

Having read Simon's case study, reflect on your knowledge-base and what is needed to support him post-surgery and through his ongoing problems. Next, identify what you know and how you know it is evidence-based and critically discuss this with a qualified nurse. If there is anything you don't know, identify what it is.

An outline of what you might include is provided at the end of this chapter.

Like Simon, many patients you care for will have more than one healthcare problem. As you learnt in Chapter 1, you work as part of a multidisciplinary team (MDT) whose collective knowledge would help to support Simon. You won't necessarily know everything about all Simon's health needs, but you do need to know to whom you can refer him, to ensure you can collectively provide the best (evidence-based) care for Simon.

Sources of evidence

To provide evidence-based care, you need to know how to access the best evidence available. At a simple level, evidence can be divided into two sources. The first is called *primary* data, which is where you go out and collect data yourself: through research, audit, or a service evaluation. You wouldn't normally undertake primary research as a nursing associate, but you will participate in audit (NMC, 2018b). We will discuss primary research more in the next chapter and audit and service evaluation in the final chapter of this book.

The other type is called *secondary* data. This is where you look at evidence (research/audit/ service evaluations or any other source other than your own primary data) that other people have carried out, written or told you about, that you then use to inform your own practice. When seeking knowledge that would help you care for Simon (see case study above) you will likely have identified secondary data sources, such as a journal article or a specialist website. The important thing, though, is that you must be confident that your sources are reliable.

Activity 2.2　Evidence-based practice and research

When you are looking for information to help you with your clinical or course work, where do you get your information from? As well as reading primary research, you might also consider other sources of information. Below you will see a list of some possible sources. Have a look at the list and consider which are reliable and which are less so. Try to justify your answer.

- A newspaper article
- Specialist websites such as Mind
- A patient
- A nursing journal
- Social media
- NHS Choices
- Wikipedia
- A doctor
- A nurse
- Trust/organisation policies

An outline answer is provided at the end of this chapter.

With the internet being so widely available, it is all too easy to go onto the web and accept the first thing you find as the 'truth'. However, in recent years we have become more aware of 'fake' (false) news and the important need to question online information. Nevertheless, fake news is still prevalent and reminds us further of the importance of questioning what we read, particularly as fake news has been found to spread quicker than real (accurate) news (Vosoughi et al., 2018). An extreme example of this is conspiracy theory, which tends to emerge when little is known about something and when people are trying to make sense of it but feel a lack of control (UK Research and Innovation, 2021). The COVID-19 pandemic was a good example of this as it gave rise to many conspiracy theories at a time when many people spent extended periods at home, with plenty of opportunity to read about the pandemic, but not necessarily drawing on reliable sources.

Less extreme, but still important, examples are the sources that we choose to access information, both for work and for academic assignments. For instance, when you were ranking your evidence in the previous activity you may have identified social media as less reliable, thinking that it tends to be used as a means for families and friends to keep in touch and chat. However, social media platforms can also be used to follow professional groups or well-known authors in a subject in which you have a particular interest. As you'll read in the answer guide for the previous activity, this can feel like a good way of keeping up to date with information, but because you are selecting the sites and the groups that you access through interest, it can also mean that you are introducing an element of bias into what you read.

Similarly, you may have identified the doctor, or the nurse, as being 'more reliable' because of the position they hold. However, it can be easy to accept what others tell you as true, particularly if they hold a position of authority. The more power and authority a person holds, the harder we find it to challenge them (Owens, 2015). However, this doesn't always mean that what they have said is evidence-based, so it's still important to question and look at the evidence behind what you're being told. An extreme example from the news is the case of Lucy Letby, who was accused of killing three babies and attempting to kill ten others, with parents of these babies telling the court of the trust they held in Lucy at the time. Another extreme example was the surgeon Ian Patterson who was convicted of 17 accounts of 'wounding with intent' and three of 'unlawful wounding', including mastectomies on women that were later found to have been unnecessary (James, 2020).

As a nursing associate you will have a responsibility to act as an ambassador for your profession, promoting a sense of confidence for the care that you (and others) provide (NMC, 2018b). Consequently, it's important that you don't, unquestioningly, accept what others tell you is right, but both challenge and look to seek answers for yourself. Finding 'good' (unbiased) evidence sources is, therefore, important. In the next part of the chapter, we are going to explore this concept further and consider how you can identify data in an unbiased way, as well as evaluate evidence and sources of data to determine their legitimacy.

Finding reliable evidence: Database searching

As a nursing associate, you will need to search for your own evidence and use research to inform your practice (NMC, 2018b). However, there is so much literature out there that it can be difficult to know what 'good' evidence is. For example, in 1998, Wakefield published a paper in *The Lancet* which claimed a link between the MMR (measles, mumps and rubella) vaccine and autism, which was subsequently found to be fraudulent. Not only were there problems with the way he carried out the research, but he had also distorted some of the evidence, meaning that his claim of a link between the MMR vaccine and autism was later found to have been falsified (Rao and Andrade, 2011). Nevertheless, the mere suggestion of this link caused a significant rise in the number of parents who decided not to vaccinate their babies. This then saw a sharp peak in the number of cases of these diseases. Although this is another extreme example, it serves to show the importance of questioning what you read, rather than simply accepting what you are told.

It is also important that you don't simply read one paper and consider it the 'one truth'. As with the Wakefield paper, not everything you read is necessarily true. Even if the research appears to have been carried out well, the results of a study may just be down to chance. We look at this further in the following chapter. Similarly, when reading opinion pieces written by experts in the field, there are likely others that have differing opinions because they look at an issue from an alternative perspective. For example, you'll have read in the answer guide for Activity 2.2 that a sociologist might believe that nursing associates *shouldn't* wear a uniform in the acute hospital setting because it creates a barrier between them and the patient. However, an infection control nurse might argue that they *should* because of the risk of cross infection. Both perspectives are 'true' and it's important that you consider both before weighing up which you believe is the better decision.

To help you find these different perspectives, you will need to look at different types of evidence (literature) and there are different ways you might want to search for this. You might want to look for a specific paper, journal or author that you know has written about a particular subject. This is the easiest way to search, and most databases will allow you to search by title of a paper, author, or even by a particular journal. However, this might not help you broaden your understanding of a topic as you are restricting your search at the outset. Nevertheless, it can be a useful way to find a paper that you already know exists and want to read. You might want to browse and generally keep up to date with what the latest papers are saying regarding an area you have a particular interest in. This can be useful if your work focuses on a specific area of healthcare as you can set alerts to tell you when a paper, or topic, you're interested in has been published. Another way is to search for a particular topic that you want to learn more about – perhaps because you need to increase your understanding of it to write an assignment, or to help you better care for a patient in your area of practice. For this, it's important to know how to search a database and to be able to filter your results effectively.

As we've highlighted already in this chapter, it's important to steer away from 'unreliable' sources, such as a newspaper or websites aimed at patients or the general public. So where do you find *reliable* sources? Using a database is a good starting place but there are also a number to choose from, so let's run through the advantages and disadvantages of some of the main databases. Google Scholar is well known and might feel like an easy way to find what you're looking for, but try to avoid using it as it won't helpfully filter your results. For example, on the day we wrote this we used the term 'surgical stomas' into Google Scholar and it came up with 39,600 hits. Although you can narrow the search results down a little by date of publication, it doesn't allow you to do much more than that. You may then be tempted to pick out the top few to read. However, Google Scholar ranks its search results in terms of popularity (i.e. how many hits each one has had), therefore the top results are unlikely to be the most current or the most relevant. The database PubMed is better to use as it allows you to filter your results. It's also free and relatively easy to use (Greenhalgh, 2019). Most databases will require a subscription before you can access a copy of the paper you are looking for, but your university, or college, will have subscriptions so you can either use PubMed to find papers you're interested in, and then search for them through your library, or you can try to access the databases directly via your university/ college website. Certain employers (such as hospital Trusts) will have their own libraries and offer free access to databases. Many universities will also offer free use of their databases on site, so it's worth finding out the services provided at your own place of study before you qualify, so you can continue to access them afterwards.

Other databases that you might come across are MEDLINE and CINAHL which both allow you to search for articles with a nursing focus. AHMED (Allied and Complementary Medicine Databases) or PsycINFO (which include papers on mental health and behavioural sciences) might also be helpful, depending on your focus. Different databases will each use slightly different software to search for articles so it's worth searching on more than one to ensure you find all the relevant articles relating to your topic. Each database will also each work in slightly different ways, but once you've learnt the principles of doing a database search you should be able to apply them to any database you use (Coughlin and Cronin, 2021). The help function on each database is a useful starting point if you're not sure of the specific functions of any databases that you use (Hoffman et al., 2017).

Using PubMed, as an example, gives you the option of doing a basic or advanced search. Even the basic search will allow you to narrow your search down further once you've started, so you could use either. As we've seen above, just searching for the term 'surgical stoma' in a database will bring up thousands of hits and there is no way of knowing which ones will be of most use to you. Nevertheless, there are several things you can do to help refine your search to find the most relevant papers. There are a couple of easy things you can do to start. The first is to refine the search by date. If you use the Basic search option on PubMed, it will then give you additional filter options and one of these is to search by date. Ideally, your papers should be no more than five years old if they relate to practice and, otherwise, no more than ten, as in the reference we use below. The exception to this is if they are what is known as *seminal* pieces – that is, important texts that continue to be significant in their field today (Coughlan et al., 2007). Another easy starting point is to refine by English language. On PubMed you can find this option under Additional filters and then Language. There don't tend to be many papers written in other languages that will come up on your database search, but it's still worth excluding them at the start.

To help you refine your search down still further, you can use something known as 'Boolean operators'. A Boolean operator is a word, such as 'AND', 'OR' or 'NOT' that you can use to combine or exclude different key words in your search (Power, 2015). Continuing to use the term 'surgical stoma' as an example, previous research around gender issues suggested to us that it would be harder for women to cope, psychologically, with a surgical stoma, in comparison to men. Using 'surgical stoma' as a search term alone, with no other limiters, returned a result of 2,210. However, using the Advanced search option meant that we could combine a search of 'surgical stoma' 'AND' 'women'. Again, on the day we carried out our search, combining these two search terms, then limiting the search to the last five years and English-language publications reduced the number of search results to 124 hits.

Wherever you work as a nursing associate, it is likely that you will have to care for someone with a surgical stoma at some time, whatever setting you work in. However, your primary focus might be on the care you provide to your patient. There are different terms used interchangeably instead of patient, including 'service user' or 'expert by experience'. In this example you would want to search for one term OR another as any one paper will most likely just use the one term throughout. By searching for 'patient' OR 'service user' OR 'expert by experience' you will find papers that have used any of these terms.

Another example of how you might use *OR* could relate to different terms that could address the same topic. For example, the three main procedures used for a surgical stoma are: colostomy, urostomy and ileostomy (Burch, 2017), although your focus might be on people with a surgical stoma, generally, rather than any specific type. There might be articles written specifically about colostomy, urostomy or ileostomy care that are equally relevant but don't specifically mention the term, but by searching for colostomy/urostomy/ileostomy OR surgical stoma, you will find papers that have used any of these terms.

Another example still is when different spellings could be used for the same word. For example, you might specifically be interested in older adults. The term 'ageing' is spelt with an 'e' in the UK, but is spelt without an 'e' (aging) in the USA. So again, you would want to search for aging OR ageing.

Some databases will also allow you to use the Boolean term 'NOT'. You can use this when you want to exclude something from your search. For example, as in the example above, you might be interested in either colostomy *or* ileostomy but *not* urostomy. In this instance, using the Boolean operator NOT will allow you to exclude anything that isn't relevant to your search.

To summarise, the key points to consider are outlined in Table 2.1.

Table 2.1 Using Boolean operators

Boolean operator	When to use it
AND	Use AND if you want to combine two terms such as ileostomy AND surgical stoma
OR	Use OR if there are different terms to mean the same thing, such as patient OR service user OR expert by experience
	Use OR if there are different terms/words that could address the same topic, such as ileostomy OR surgical stoma
	Use OR if there are different ways of spelling the same word, such as ageing OR aging

To ensure you capture everything that is relevant it is also useful to use something called a *truncation* (Hoffman et al., 2017). This means typing in the stem of the word and then adding an Asterix. For example, using nurs* would allow you to search for hits of either nurses OR nursing.

Adding structure to your database searches

In the examples above, we started with a term that captured a vast number of hits. However, the opposite can also be true and you end up with few or no hits, or none that are relevant to what you are trying to find. For any search, the important thing to remember is to be clear about what you're searching for. Search engines work on precise terms so if you're not totally sure what you're looking for, then you can be sure that the search engine won't either. Imagine trying to describe to someone a particular item you want them to buy from the supermarket. Unless you are clear about what you want them to buy, they might come back with totally the wrong thing. A small, green, fruit could equally be an apple or a lime, for example.

To help you focus on your search, there are several tools you can use to help you structure your search. We will look at two of them here. The first tool is called PICO which stands for *population, intervention* (or *issue*), *comparison* and *outcome*, although it's also used with an 'S' on the end, standing for *studies*. This tool can be useful if you are looking for research studies (Larson et al., 2019), but can also be useful for searches generally. You don't have to use all these acronyms in your search, but they can help give your search clarity and structure. Table 2.2 below gives an example of how it could be used.

Another you could use is the PCC tool (Peters et al., 2020). This stands for *population, concept, context* (or who, what and where). It can be used if you are looking for general papers on a topic you don't know much about, although it uses similar ideas to the PICO(S) tool above, so you will see some overlap. Table 2.3 gives an example of how it could be used.

Table 2.2 Using the PICO(S) tool

Population (P)	Identify all the different terms (called a MeSH term in PubMed) (Foster, 2015) that could be used to describe your particular population of interest
	You can also use this section to consider the setting your population is in, if it's relevant to your search. For example, if you were interested in people with a surgical stoma, you might specifically be interested in those who are being cared for in care homes
Intervention or issue (I)	An intervention is a 'thing' that you use or do. Examples of this could be a type of dressing (something you use) or turning of a patient in bed (something you do). You would use an issue when not much is known about a subject and you want to learn more about it. This is particularly helpful when considering the experiences of those you care for – for example, older women living with a stoma
	In terms of research, if the focus is on an intervention then the research will be quantitative. If the focus is on an issue then the research will be qualitative. We will discuss different types of research in the next chapter
Comparison (C)	This is normally only used when searching for research that compares one intervention to another, so wouldn't be relevant to the examples we've used so far
Outcome (O)	You may or may not want to narrow down your search further by including an outcome, but this could be used to further focus your search. For example, in research it can be used as a measure of effectiveness for whether the intervention works or not. Examples could be a reduction in hospital admissions or a reduction in symptoms. Other examples could include mortality rates, readmission rates or levels of health-related complications (to name a few), depending on the focus of the topic
Studies (S)	Again, this relates more to research studies but can also be useful to consider the types of articles you want to include. For example, are you only interested in research studies and, if so, what types (qualitative or quantitative)? Or are you considering other types of papers, such as opinion or theoretical articles?
	In this section, we also tend to include our date limiters, i.e. if we're only focusing on the last five years, or whatever dates are relevant to the topic of our focus

Table 2.3 Using the PCC tool

Population (P)	The population in this example relates just to the group of people you are interested in. This could be broad such as 'women' or more specific, such as 'women with a surgical stoma'
Concept (C)	The concept is the issue or the topic that you're interested in. This could be an intervention or an issue, but equally it could be that you want to focus on the outcome
Context (C)	The context refers to the setting in which you're interested. For example, you might want to focus just on care homes, rather than the hospital setting

It might feel a little overwhelming when you first start, but the best way to learn how to do something is to have a go.

Activity 2.3   Research

Using the PICO(S) tool, consider all the terms you could use to find articles relevant to people with a surgical stoma, living in a care home. Remember you don't have to use all the sections and, in our basic example, it wouldn't be appropriate to do so, but it will hopefully help you build your confidence in using the tool. Next, have a go at using the PCC tool to consider the experiences of women living with a surgical stoma.

An outline answer is given at the end of this chapter.

Undertaking a database search may seem complicated at first, but it is a skill that will improve the more you use it. It is worth making time to practise it, to ensure you are able to read both deeply and widely around your topic area in a systematic way.

Chapter summary

This chapter builds on what you learnt in Chapter 1 and acts as a building block to the learning activities you will cover in Chapter 3 and beyond. To provide good-quality healthcare you must ensure your care is evidence-based. We started with a case study to help you consider what evidence you might need to provide this care, and some examples of specialist websites you might use to help build up your knowledge of this particular condition. We used the essence of Simon's health condition as a theme throughout but link this to different genders, age groups and settings to show how the principles apply across different care settings and patient groups that a nursing associate may experience. We then considered the different types of evidence and what to use – or avoid using – when selecting what to read. Finally, we looked at how to find literature and ways to search for literature, systematically. Working towards becoming a nursing associate is just the beginning of your journey into life-long learning. Whether you decide to remain as a nursing associate, or continue to study further, you will be expected to ensure your practice is evidence-based. Practising the skills identified in this chapter will help you to achieve this in a structured and systematic way.

Activities: Brief outline answers

Activity 2.1 Critical thinking and reflection

Simon has complex, long-term health needs. In caring for Simon, you will want to ensure you understand his conditions and health needs. In summary these are:

- sub-total colectomy
- ulcerative colitis

- ulcerative colitis flare-up
- pain management
- stoma
- the practicalities of living with a stoma
- how to empty, clean and change an ileostomy bag
- how to order ileostomy bags
- the psychological/emotional impact of having an ileostomy
- diet, nutrition and vitamin D deficiency
- vitamin D indications and contra-indications
- steroid indications and contra-indications – especially when taken over a long period
- total proctocolectomy.

This chapter discusses how best to find evidence relating to this condition and consider specific conditions relevant to your own practice and setting. Reflecting on your own level of knowledge is important too as it will help establish your baseline of understanding and whether or not that understanding is evidence-based and the evidence is relevant to you as a nursing associate, or is aimed at the general public (we cover that further in Activity 2.2). As well as secondary sources we cover in this chapter, it is worth looking at specialist websites such as those below. Some will be aimed at the general public but many (as in those included here) also have sections specifically aimed at healthcare professionals:

- Colostomy UK (www.colostomyuk.org/),
- Crohn's and Colitis UK (www.crohnsandcolitis.org.uk/)
- Crohn's and Colitis Foundation (www.crohnscolitisfoundation.org/)

NICE will also produce guidelines on most conditions. Here is a link to what they say regarding the management of ulcerative colitis: www.nice.org.uk/guidance/ng130

Your Trust/organisational policies are generally based on NICE guidelines so you should also look to see what they say.

The World Health Organization (WHO) (www.who.int/) is also a useful resource for up-to-date guidance on a whole range of healthcare practices and conditions.

You may also want to consider the common health conditions you come across in your own area of practice. Have a look to see what specialist websites are available that relate to these.

You should aim to *triangulate* the evidence that you read (i.e. not just rely on one source). This will not only help you ensure you gain a wide range of information, but also ensure that the evidence you read is more likely to be reliable.

Don't forget, too, that the patient and (where appropriate) their family are important resources. Everyone is unique and will experience their condition individually. They will know best of all how *they* feel and what works best for them.

Activity 2.2 Evidence-based practice and research

Here are some of the things you should consider:

A newspaper article

Newspapers report what others have done. They tend to be biased and often have a particular political slant, so they are not reliable. The broadsheets can help you to identify current issues of interest, but you should always look for the original research paper and read that rather than relying simply on what the newspaper says.

Specialist websites such as Mind

Specialist websites can be a useful way of gaining up-to-date information about a specific topic, particularly if you don't know much about it. The websites listed in Activity 2.1, for example, all have sections aimed at professionals. However, Mind is aimed at people experiencing mental health problems and doesn't have a section for healthcare professionals. Reading information aimed at non-professionals can be a useful way of helping you gain some understanding of the topic, but you should always use it as a stepping-stone to move on to resources that are aimed at professionals as these will explain and explore issues in greater depth, and are more likely to be evidence- rather than experience-based.

A patient

As you learnt in Chapter 1, listening to the patient is always important as they are experts in their own right (and thus can also be known as experts by experience). Two people with an identical health condition might experience it in different ways. Working *with* patients, therefore, is important. Your role will be to offer advice and guidance on the best evidence available to help them make an informed decision, and to signpost them to appropriate services.

A nursing journal

There are a wide variety of nursing journals available and some will rank higher than others. The quality of the journal tends to be gauged by something known as its *impact factor* which is calculated by the number of times someone cites that paper in another journal. The higher the impact factor the 'better' the journal is considered – and the harder it is to get a paper published as they have stringent quality measures, including a system of *peer review* (a peer, who is an expert on the subject area, checks the quality of a paper before it's published). Primary studies are the best to read, but an opinion piece by a well-known author in their field is also worth reading. No nursing journal has a high impact factor, but the *British Journal of Nursing*, for example, is higher than the *Nursing Standard*, although both peer review their articles.

Social media (including blogs)

Surprisingly not all social media is, necessarily, bad. Following a well-known author in their field on X (formerly Twitter), for example, can help you stay up to date with their recent publications. They can also signpost you to other useful authors that you might want to read. There is an important caveat to this, however. The problem with following someone you are interested in is that it could mean that you get a biased view on a topic. As a nursing associate it's important that you can give a balanced view on an issue and this means understanding it from different perspectives. For example, if you were asked if nursing associates should wear a uniform in the acute hospital setting you might answer 'yes'. However, could you also argue why they shouldn't? From a sociological perspective, you might argue that it causes a barrier between yourself and the patient. You might also argue that other professionals (such as some doctors) don't wear a uniform. However, if you were to consider it from the perspective of an infection control nurse, then you would weigh up all these arguments but still decide that 'yes', wearing a uniform is important. Again, reading widely about a topic will help you develop a balanced understanding of an issue.

NHS Choices

As you'll have read earlier, this resource can be a good place to start looking as it will give you a basic insight into an issue. However, it is aimed at the general public and, as a future healthcare professional, you need to have more insight into an issue than the general public requires. So, there's nothing wrong with starting here, but only to give you a basic understanding. Then go on to read sources aimed at healthcare professionals.

Wikipedia

There is a lot of rhetoric about Wikipedia and that it is unreliable. Interestingly, Wikipedia itself highlights the fact that anyone can edit its information. Normally, your lecturers won't want you to be citing it for this reason. However, as with the NHS Choices website, it can be a useful starting point to gain a bit of knowledge about a subject, before moving on to texts that are more reliable and in-depth.

A doctor

Other healthcare professionals can be useful sources of knowledge, especially if they have specialised in a particular area. However, as we highlighted in Chapter 1, it is easy to be in awe of a doctor and therefore accept what they say as 'true'. It's important you still check the evidence for yourself. When you are a registered nursing associate you will be accountable for the decisions you make and must ensure these are informed and not purely based on the word of another professional. As a trainee nursing associate your lecturers will also want to see you develop decision-making skills based on evidence, so you will need to show your views come from reading the evidence for yourself.

A nurse

Like doctors, nurses can also be a good source of information, but you mustn't just accept what they tell you as the 'one truth'. As you gain experience from different practice areas you might find that what is considered 'best practice' in one area is not in another. This can cause confusion as to which one is best. Again, this is the reason why you must read deeply and widely around the topic area.

Trust/organisation policies

Your Trust/organisational policies will be research- and evidence-based and provide a good source for evidence-based healthcare. Often, they will come from NICE guidelines.

Wherever you find information, it's important not to rely on just one source. Even if it is a research paper that has been published in a journal with a high impact factor, there might be flaws in the way the research was carried out (as we'll discuss in the next chapter), or their results might be down to chance. We call consulting multiple sources the triangulation of evidence. In addition, your lecturers will want to see that you have drawn on a variety of sources to support your work to ensure you are well informed.

Activity 2.3 Research

PICO(S) and PCC

The important thing is to include as much detail as you can in each of the sections. For example, there are several conditions where someone would have a surgical stoma and it's important to list all of them. Similarly, there are different terms that can mean care home. As you start to search it's likely you will discover new terms you'd not considered before, so should also add these to your search terms.

Population (P)	Surgical stoma
	Stoma
	Intestinal stoma
	Colostomy
	Urostomy
	Ileostomy
	Care home
	Nursing home
	Residential home
Intervention/issue (I)	Stoma care
	Ostomy care
	Colostomy care
	Urostomy care
	Ileostomy care
Comparison (C)	No search terms included here as it wasn't relevant to the search topic
Outcome (O)	No search terms included here either but if you wanted to focus on something specific then you would include it here
Studies (S)	Primary research papers (normally you would break this down into types of research and we'll look at this in more detail in the next chapter)
	Theoretical pieces
	Opinion pieces
	Restricted to the last five years
	Written in English

Here's what you might include for the second example using the PCC tool, focusing on women with a surgical stoma:

Population (P)	Woman
	Women
	Female
	Females
Concept (C)	Stoma
	Surgical stoma
	Ostomy
	Colostomy
	Urostomy
	Ileostomy

Context (C)	Stoma care
	Surgical stoma care
	Ostomy care
	Colostomy care
	Urostomy care
	Ileostomy care

Annotated further reading

Ellis, P (2023) *Evidence Based Practice in Nursing* (5th edition). London: Learning Matters.

This book is aimed at nurses, generally, and also focuses on different types of evidence that nurses can and do use in practice.

Greasley, P (2016) *Doing Essays and Assignments: Essential Tips for Students* (2nd edition). London: Sage.

Chapter 5 of this book is entitled 'Reading and researching the literature' and is written as a series of 'tips'. The chapter includes a more detailed discussion than in this chapter as to why not to use Wikipedia as a source of evidence as well as further information on carrying out a literature search. The book isn't specifically written for nurses, or nursing associates, but many of the examples used relate to healthcare.

Useful websites

https://pubmed.ncbi.nlm.nih.gov/

This is the PubMed website that is used within this chapter. At the bottom of the page there are useful links to additional information and guides to help you with your searches.

https://paperpile.com/g/research-databases-healthcare/

This website provides an overview of different databases, specific for articles relevant to healthcare, that you could use for your database search, listing the pros and cons for each.

www.rcn.org.uk/library/Support/Literature-searching-and-training/How-to-undertake-a-literature-search

This website is created by the RCN and includes useful short videos on the different elements of undertaking a literature search. The videos include searching through the RCN, CINAHL and the British Nursing Index (BNI) databases and give useful examples of using different databases, other than PubMed. The examples include many of the filtering processes covered in this chapter. We didn't include the RCN database in the chapter as you have to be a member of the RCN to use it, but this section of the site is available to all.

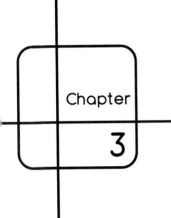

Chapter 3

Understanding research

Melissa Owens

Chapter aims

After reading this chapter you will be able to:

* understand the importance of primary research;
* understand the difference between quantitative and qualitative research designs;
* appreciate how different research designs would be used to understand different phenomena;
* appreciate the importance of ethics in carrying out primary research;
* understand the contribution that service users can play in ensuring research designs are fit for purpose.

Introduction

As highlighted in Chapters 1 and 2, the NMC Code (2018a) requires nurses and nursing associates to 'practise effectively'. We introduced this theme to you in Chapters 1 and 2 by, first, getting you to think about what constitutes evidence and, second, by providing you with the opportunity to carry out a database search using recognised tools and databases. In this chapter, we focus on the role of primary research and how to make sense of it to inform your practice. We guide you to build on the knowledge you have gained so far, by introducing you to the principles of research and different research designs and what they are used for, with structured activities to support your learning.

We have found some nurses and nursing associates to have an inexplicable fear of anything that involves the term 'research'. However, as with anything you learn, it's important to find a text that makes sense of the topic, for you, and is written at a level that you understand. We have tried to write this chapter in such a way as to achieve these two goals, with activities that build up your knowledge and understanding sequentially. However, we have only been able to provide an introduction to the topic here and it's important that you read around the topic in more detail. We have, therefore, suggested further reading and website resources at the end of the chapter to help you build up your knowledge, understanding and confidence further.

Making sense of research

First, we need to bust a myth. Research is *not* all about people in white coats doing experiments in laboratories. It can be, but for you as a nursing associate it's more relevant to think of it as a means of ensuring that what you do in practice is both evidence-based *and* best practice. The Code (NMC, 2018a) tells you that you must 'practise effectively' and in line with the *best* evidence that is available. If you simply follow the instructions given to you by a doctor or a nurse, how can you be sure it is based on the *best* evidence? In effect, you can't. As we discussed in Chapter 1, as a nursing associate you are accountable for what you do, so you must ensure it is correct.

Conversely, simply reading one research paper and basing, or changing, your practice on that, also isn't enough. As you will have read in the previous chapter, some research studies are conducted badly, or can even falsify their results, as in the case of Wakefield's 1998 study (see Chapter 2) claiming a link between the MMR vaccine and autism. As nursing associates, it is important that you develop critical skills that enable you to evaluate whether a piece of research is credible or not. To do so, you must be able to understand the different types of research designs and how they *should* be carried out, so that you can judge for yourself how much confidence you can have in their results. Once you have grasped this, you will then be able to recognise if and where there are flaws in their design that might impact on their conclusions. We will introduce you to the principles of critiquing research in the following chapter.

To help you make sense of how research relates to the health of those for whom you care, we have created a case study which we will refer to throughout this chapter and to which we will link some of the principles of the research designs and methodologies that we discuss. Have a read of the case scenario now.

Case study: Toni (Part 1)

Toni is a 13-year-old adolescent who identifies as transgender but was born female. Toni uses the pronoun 'he'. Toni is currently struggling with anxiety, for which he has been prescribed Sertraline 50mg. He is also overweight.

Toni lives in Bradford, with his parents, and attends the local secondary school, which he dislikes; he often tells of feeling isolated. Toni has one close friend, Sarah, that he spends much of his free time with. Toni is also close to his grandmother, who lives close by.

When Toni was born, his parents were approached and asked if they would take part in a large research study called 'Born in Bradford', to which they agreed.

Three weeks ago, Toni fractured his ankle and is currently non-weight bearing.

Activity 3.1   Research

We will return to Toni throughout this chapter but there are a few things we want you to do before that.

First, read the following paper: GATE (2023) *Reaffirming Autonomy of Trans and Gender Diverse Children and Adolescents*, https://gate.ngo/wp-content/uploads/2023/07/Reaffirming-autonomy-of-TGD-Children-and-Adolescents.pdf to help you appreciate the global issues identified for young trans people.

There is no outline answer at the end of the chapter.

If you have difficulty finding this, or any other paper in this chapter (or indeed this book), then ask your librarian to help you. This first article should be readily available by copying and pasting the link into a web browser. Others, however, should all be available by doing a database search using the skills you learnt in Chapter 2. However, some organisations subscribe to different journals than others so it isn't possible to say how easily *everyone* will be able to access any particular paper. Just a word of warning: if you go straight to the site of an online journal without being logged in to an organisational account (your university, college, Trust) it might ask you to pay a large sum of money to purchase the article. **Don't do it!** If you genuinely can't get hold of any article, we suggest there are two things you can do.

1.   You can order any article via an 'Interlibrary Loan', through a university or college library for a very small amount of money and they will get it for you fairly quickly.
2.   If you are using this book as part of a module you are studying then ask your module leader to get the papers and add them to your online module reading list. They can order them and make them available for everyone taking your module.

Now let's return to the focus of our chapter and have a go at Activity 3.2.

Activity 3.2   Critical thinking

Consider what you think these terms mean. An explanation of each is provided in more detail below.

- Quantitative
- Deductive
- Qualitative
- Inductive

Quantitative research

Even if you weren't sure of the answer, hopefully you could make a good guess from the words themselves. *Quantitative research*, for example, has 'quant' as its stem which can be short for quantity, or quantifiable. Another way to remember this is to think of quantity as a set of numbers. Quantitative research refers to research which collects and analyses numerical data. It's perhaps the definition you think of first when asked to consider the meaning of research because, as we said earlier, it *can* mean people in white coats in a laboratory recording measurements and data, but it also relates to any research carried out in a certain way – that is, deductively.

Deductive

From the term 'deductive' you might have identified that the stem of this is to *deduce* – that is, to work out. If you watch detective series on television, you may have seen the detective follow a systematic process to get to the 'single truth' and come to a conclusion as to who killed X. You might then watch the court drama play out, where the jury are told they must establish 'beyond reasonable doubt' if the person on trial actually killed X. In essence, they follow a *deductive* approach in order to prove, or disprove, something.

Quantitative research works in a similar way, with researchers drawing their conclusions in a controlled and scientific manner in order to reach the 'one truth'. To continue with the court-room analogy, either the defendant is 'guilty' or 'not guilty'. Applying this principle to quantitative research: either it works or it doesn't/it's right or it's wrong/it's good or it's bad, as this type of research generally deals with things that are concrete and absolute (i.e. they are *binary*).

Activity 3.3   Critical thinking

You plant a sunflower in your garden and tend it, lovingly, for several weeks until, in August, it reaches its full height and is 15 feet tall.

Your neighbour also planted a sunflower in their garden and tended it, lovingly, for several weeks. However, when they measure their sunflower in August it is only 6 feet tall.

Why might they be so different in height?

An outline answer is provided at the end of this chapter.

When reading quantitative research papers you will find that many will describe their research as having followed a specific research design. Others won't, but will follow the *principles* of a deductive (quantitative) approach. Let's look at a paper that is deductive in its approach.

Activity 3.4   Research

Use the database searching skills you learnt in the previous chapter to find, and then read, the following research paper. By reading the answer guide to Activity 3.3 above, you will have gleaned a little knowledge of the technical terms you might come across in quantitative research. However, don't worry, at this stage, about trying to understand any more of the technical terms that they use, as you should be able to follow *what* they did without necessarily understanding the specifics of *how* they did it.

Pistella, J, Ioverno, S, Rodgers, M and Russell, S (2020) The contribution of school safety to weight-related health behaviours for transgender youth. *Journal of Adolescence*, 78: 33–42

This is the first of four papers we will ask you to find in this chapter.

Often in quantitative, deductive research papers, the authors tell you, the reader, what their theories were (i.e. what they believed the results of their research would be) before they carried out their research.

1. What are the theories that the authors tell you?
2. How might the results of this paper help you better understand why Toni, the teenager in our case scenario, is overweight?

An outline of what you might include is provided at the end of this chapter.

It's important to remember that this study only looked at eating behaviours associated with schooling and that Toni, our youth in the case scenario, also had a diagnosed mental health condition, which this study didn't consider. Reading one research paper, therefore, might only give you one piece of a jigsaw and you will need to read other papers to help you get a fuller understanding.

Pistella et al.'s (2020) research, clearly used a deductive approach. However, while they started with particular theories that they believed to be true, what they found by the end of their study was that their theories weren't necessarily true, and it was more complex and messy than they had originally thought.

There are many types of research that are carried out, using deductive reasoning, but they will all still follow the same principles, which are illustrated in Figure 3.1 below.

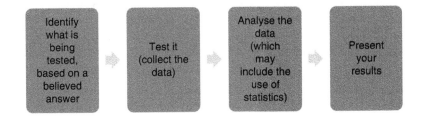

Figure 3.1 The principles of research using quantitative research

Let's go through three common research designs.

Randomised control trial (RCT) (also known as an 'experimental study')

This is probably the most well-known type of research and, even if you haven't heard of it before, you will most likely be familiar with the process. An RCT compares one thing against another and attempts to control (thus the name) the variables (anything that could affect the results of the trial) as far as possible.

To do this the researchers will select a 'sample' (of people) that is representative of the population under study. They are then 'randomly' (thus the name) divided into two groups. One is given the intervention being studied and the other a different intervention or a placebo. In its purest form the researchers won't know which group is given the intervention and which isn't, but this does depend on what is being tested. If it's a drug, for example, this could be easily disguised so that no one knows which is which. If it is a therapeutic intervention (for example, group cognitive behavioural therapy (CBT) versus one-to-one CBT) or a tool to measure pain (for example, the Visual Analogue Scale versus the Numerical Rating Scale) then this wouldn't be possible.

The intervention is provided in a controlled way that prevents anything else, as far as possible, affecting the outcome. For example, if you wanted to study the effect of an antidepressant drug then you would need to ensure that any results were conclusively due to the effect of the drug and not due to anything else. For example, if someone was taking an antidepressant drug and undertaking CBT, you wouldn't know which, if either, was the one having any effect.

The effect of the intervention is then observed over a period of time (the data are collected) and the results analysed, normally through statistical analysis. This type of research is considered the 'gold standard' of research as it tends to involve a large sample carried out in a controlled way that eliminates the possibility of any bias ('variables') influencing the results. Commonly associated with drug trials, it can also be used to test many interventions you will be familiar with and have used as a nursing associate.

You may also find different variations of these designs. For example: an RCT where neither the researcher nor the participants know if they are getting the intervention or not (for example, in a drug trial where there is a placebo used as a comparison), is known as a *double-blinded RCT*. Another example is if one group receives the intervention and then swaps with the group who didn't (which is known as a *crossover RCT*).

Activity 3.5   Critical thinking

Toni, from our earlier case study, takes Sertraline. All drugs are tested using RCTs. Consider what common interventions, or tools, you use in your practice. Which of these do you think were originally tested by RCT? I've suggested four in the paragraph above (group CBT versus one-to-one CBT; and Visual Analogue Scale versus the Numerical Rating Scale).

As this is based on your own practice, there is no outline answer provided at the end of this chapter.

Not all research can be carried out by an RCT and, for many different types of studies, it wouldn't be ethical to do so either (we'll look at the principle of ethics later in this chapter, and in Chapter 6).

Cohort study (also known as a 'non-experimental study')

A cohort study is an example of a study you would carry out if you are not able to use an RCT to find your answer. Cohort studies tend to be made up of a large sample and are generally studied prospectively (looking forward in time) with a sample (group of people) who share a similar characteristic, or a risk factor, compared to another that do not.

In the case study above, we told you that Toni and his family were part of a research study called 'Born in Bradford' (BiB). BiB is a cohort study which involved studying families who gave birth to children in the city of Bradford (so, in this instance, for Toni, being born in Bradford is the shared characteristic or risk factor that he has in common with others in the study). Previous studies had identified a high level of childhood illnesses in children born in Bradford, in comparison to those born in other deprived cities, and this study attempts to explore the reasons behind it.

Activity 3.6   Critical thinking

Have a look at the website for the BiB project and specifically the section on the BiB family cohort: https://borninbradford.nhs.uk/what-we-do/cohort-studies/bib-family-cohort/to help you get an insight into what a cohort study might look like

What different data collection methods do they use for this study?

An outline answer is available at the end of the chapter.

Case control study

A notable difference between a cohort study and a case control study is that a cohort study will look *forward* in time to find similarities between people who share the same characteristic or risk. In a case control study, the researchers look *back*, retrospectively, to look at a sample of people who already have a condition or disease, to observe what risk factors they shared that may have contributed to their development of a condition (the cases) in comparison to those who don't (the control).

A well-known, historical example of a case control study is from the outbreak of a fatal condition in cattle known as 'mad cow disease' (the official name for this was Bovine spongiform encephalopathy) in the 1980s, which then spread to humans (called Creutzfeldt-Jakob disease) and caused a widespread fear across the country at that time. Scientists didn't initially know what was causing the condition and had to look back in time to identify what the animals (and then the humans) might share as risk factors to cause them to have developed this condition.

Other types of quantitative research

Many other studies that you read might not tell you what type of research study design they used, as in the paper by Pistella et al. (2020) that we asked you to read earlier. This is often the case if the researchers follow the principles of quantitative research, but their research doesn't fit into a specific research design, such as those described above. A common example of this is when the study is small and the researchers want feedback on something specific, using a questionnaire or survey. An example of this that you might have been involved in, could be a questionnaire you are asked to complete at the end of a module you've studied. Normally, there is a set of questions to answer 'yes/no' or 'agree/disagree'. While there may be an opportunity to add 'free text' comments, the specific questions themselves cannot be altered and it is these that allow your tutors to add up how many learners gave one answer over another to gauge if there was anything they needed to do differently when they deliver their module again.

Qualitative research

Hopefully you were also able to make a good guess at the meaning of this term, with the stem being *qual* which should make you think of *quality*. Qualitative research is often described as being the opposite of all things related to quantitative research. This is perhaps a generalisation, but the origins of qualitative research stem from a rejection of quantitative research and its relevance to some disciplines (and, in particular, health and healthcare). Qualitative research concerns itself with collecting and analysing non-numerical data, and using it to understand attitudes, opinions, experiences or other phenomena that can't be easily quantified.

It is a useful starting point to understanding what qualitative research involves. Sometimes, learners will (wrongly) try to apply the *principles* of quantitative research to that of qualitative research, because that is what they believe research should look like. However, qualitative research is very different to quantitative research, and that's why it's helpful to think of quantitative and qualitative research as being opposites. We will try to explain this further in the examples given below.

Activity 3.7   Critical thinking

Read the following paper: Medico, D, Sansfaçon, A, Zufferey, A, Galantino, G, Bosom, M and Suerich-Gulick, F (2020) Pathways to gender affirmation in trans-youth: A qualitative and participative study with youth and their parents. *Clinical Child Psychology and Psychiatry*, 25(4): 1002–1014.

As with the Pistella et al. (2020) paper that we first asked you to read in this chapter, this article doesn't align itself to any particular methodology, but describes itself as 'qualitative' and should help you appreciate the general *principles* of qualitative research. Once you've read it, identify the key ways in which the researchers carried out their research and how they differ from those identified in the Pistella et al. (2020) study.

An outline answer is provided at the end of this chapter.

Inductive

The term 'inductive' means that the researcher wants to explore something (a 'phenomenon') they don't believe they know the answer to or want to understand further. They, therefore, investigate the phenomena in depth, looking for patterns, in order to draw conclusions. Figure 3.2 attempts to outline the process by which qualitative research is carried out (inductively) to help you see how it differs from that of quantitative research.

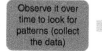 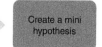

Figure 3.2   The principles of research using qualitative research

Although we've presented this as a linear process, it actually isn't. Researchers will begin to analyse their data as soon as they start to collect it, using this to help them create a mini hypothesis which they then test out by collecting further data. This process continues until the researcher is confident they have enough data to draw reliable conclusions.

Another, significant, difference between quantitative and qualitative research is that qualitative researchers are a key part of the data-gathering process. As we explained above, in quantitative research, the researcher tries to isolate the 'thing' being studied so they can be sure the results are directly due to the intervention. Consequently, they will try to distance themselves from what is being studied – metaphorically, putting 'it' into a sterile box. This comes from the theory that everything should be measurable and testable (i.e. it can be studied under scientific conditions). In qualitative research, researchers are interested in the *complexities* of life, and therefore look at all that is happening, rather than one isolated, sterile factor. As such they are an integral part of the data collection process. They will ask questions, reflect on the answers, often keep a reflective journal, consider what to explore next – who they want to talk to, look at, read about – in order to help them gain a better understanding of the phenomena under study.

It is worth pointing out that qualitative researchers often also reject some of the terminology used by quantitative researchers and the use of the term 'phenomena' is a good example of this. Quantitative researchers often describe what they are investigating as a 'problem'. In qualitative research, however, what is being investigated isn't necessarily a problem and, therefore, different terms tend to be used instead. This can make understanding all the different terms confusing at times. To help you understand some of the common terminology you might read, we've created Table 3.1, which includes some of the different terminologies you might come across in quantitative and qualitative research.

Table 3.1   Quantitative and qualitative research terminology

Term	Meaning
Research design	All quantitative research has general principles in common, but the bigger studies will also use a particular framework, such as an RCT, cohort study or case control study. The collective term for this is 'research design'
Variables	Sometimes written as *independent variables*, these are anything that could affect the outcome of a quantitative study that isn't part of what the researcher wants to test
Causation	This is generally associated with an RCT and means that something directly *causes* something else to happen
Correlation	This means that although something else is happening at the same time, it doesn't mean one thing necessarily caused the other
Hypothesis	This is used in RCTs, specifically, instead of a research question and is a statement used to predict what the result of an experiment will be
Research methodology	All qualitative research has general principles in common but, in the same way as quantitative research, many will use a particular framework. Whereas in quantitative research this is collectively known as the research design, in qualitative research, it can be known as the 'research methodology'
Saturation	A term used in qualitative research to mean the point at which the researcher is confident they have collected sufficient data to be able to draw reliable conclusions

This list isn't exhaustive, however, so it's a good idea to make your own list each time you come across a new term, to help you remember it.

Subjectivity and objectivity

Qualitative research is also interested in the *subjective*, the experiences of people and how they interact with the world, either consciously or subconsciously. Qualitative researchers reject the 'one truth' (the metaphorical sterile box) view of the world that is rational and orderly and aims to be *objective*. Instead, they want to find a way to understand how people *experience* their worlds.

Even if you have not yet had to break bad news to someone, it is likely that at some time you will have to. When you do you could find that the way in which you give that news will make a difference to how they respond to it – that is, there is no one truth to someone's experiences. To give another example: if you feel upset by a comment someone makes, the person who upset you can't then say that your reaction is wrong; or that you are not feeling how you say you feel. Feelings are individual and subjective to whatever is going on around you. This feeling cannot be identified as a 'problem' that is then isolated and tested. Qualitative research is interested in this subjective, experiential way in which people interact with, and respond to, the world in which they live and is, therefore, carried out *inductively*.

As with the examples for quantitative research, we've provided a description below of three common methodologies. However, there are many others and the number continues to grow every day.

Phenomenology

Phenomenology is one of the commonest methodologies used in nursing. Although there are two types of phenomenology that you might come across, both focus on the *experiences* of people and the meaning given to it by those who experience it, rather than that of the researcher.

Think, for example, about how you feel when you stand on the beach and look at the sea. If you are a confident swimmer, you might find this a positive experience and feel like you want to go towards the water. However, someone who is nervous of the sea, or perhaps has had a bad experience in the water, may feel very differently. You can see from this example how a qualitative, phenomenological approach might help the researcher understand people's experiences better.

To give an example in relation to healthcare: it might be used to better understand how people come to terms with a life-threatening, or inhibiting, condition. In phenomenology, data are generally collected by interviewing participants using a set of open-ended questions to encourage participants to open up and talk. These questions could change and be adapted as they discover, or want to discover, more. These are then transcribed into written text. Analysis then takes place by reading and rereading the data, looking for themes and connections made between the different transcripts. Researchers will often keep a diary as they collect data to help them reflect on their data and understand it at a deeper level.

Activity 3.8   Critical analysis and reflection

Use the database searching skills you learnt in the previous chapter to find, and read, the following article.

Roach, A, Thomas, S, Abdoli, S, Wright, M and Yates, A (2021) Kids helping kids: The lived experience of adolescents who support friends with mental health needs. *Journal of Child Adolescent Psychiatry Nursing*, 34: 32–40

Again, there will most likely be words used in this article that you're not familiar with, but don't worry about these too much now. The meaning of the article should be clear enough without having to look up the words.

Returning to our case scenario, Toni struggled with anxiety. Having read this article, what impact do you now think might Toni's anxiety have had on his friend, Sarah?

Now consider your own area of practice. How might this article help you to understand the burden of caring better in relation to your own practice?

An outline of what you might include is provided at the end of this chapter.

Ethnography

You may have heard of the concept of *anthropology* whereby historical researchers took themselves off to distant lands to learn about Indigenous populations by living with them for an extended period of time. Ethnography bases itself on this concept, but, instead of distant populations, it focuses on those closer to home: subcultures within our own cultures. Examples relating to healthcare could be the care experienced in a hospice, or a care home, or an acute psychiatric setting. Researchers then spend time in this setting observing what is going on.

In this type of research, the researcher is interested in the behaviours and practices of the group – that is, their *culture*, rather than the meaning people place on their experiences. Therefore, researchers will look for beliefs, values and shared meanings of those within the subculture under study and particularly those that are taken for granted or carried out subconsciously.

In ethnography, data can be collected in a number of ways, but often it is done through the researcher immersing themselves into the subculture they are exploring and asking questions of participants, informally, when questions arise. However, many methods of data collection can be used which help the researcher explore what is happening in their field of study. Some of these could include undertaking interviews with key stakeholders and reviewing documentation. As with phenomenology, the researcher will analyse their data as they go along, reading and rereading it and keeping a diary to aid their understanding.

A classic example of an ethnographic study is the work of Goffman who published his work on 'asylums' in 1961. Ethically (we look at ethics in more detail later), health researchers are no longer permitted to go 'undercover' to do their research, but this isn't always the case in social research. At the time, it allowed Goffman to work as an assistant to a physical education instructor without others knowing his true reason for being there – which was to study, in depth, the functioning of a mental health institution at that time. His description of the power relations between staff and patients is strongly believed to have influenced the closure of mental health institutions across the western world (Adlam et al., 2013).

Activity 3.9   Critical thinking and reflection

Again, use the database searching skills that you learnt in the previous chapter to find, and then read, the following article.

McGlashan, H and Fitzpatrick, K (2018) I use any pronouns, and I'm questioning everything else: Transgender youth and the issue of gender pronouns. *Sex Education*, 18(3): 239–252

Now answer the following questions.

- How might your reading of this article have increased your understanding of why Toni felt isolated at school?
- What policies are in place in your own workplace to care for people who identify as transgender?
- What might you do differently, in practice, having read this article?

An outline answer is provided at the end of this chapter.

Grounded theory research

Grounded theory research is the third common type of qualitative research that we want to introduce you to in this chapter. It was originally created by American researchers Glaser and Strauss in 1967 as a way of generating new theories, as opposed to proving (or disproving) existing ones (Cooney, 2010) that are *grounded* in (come from) the data.

Grounded theorists focus on groups of people who have shared (common) experiences. However, there are various different approaches to grounded theory that have evolved over time with the commonest created by the leading proponents of grounded theory, Glaser and Strauss, Glaser alone, Strauss alone and, most recently, by Charmaz. What each has in common is that they use a highly structured approach to collecting and analysing data and focus on 'something' where little is known about the subject being studied at the start and ends with a new theory being proposed. Unlike other qualitative methodologies, it is a 'total' approach whereby the researcher is guided through the whole research process, using a structured (grounded theory) framework.

As was highlighted earlier, qualitative research tends to collect and analyse data simultaneously and this approach was first used in grounded theory to aid the development of ideas and direct them towards what further data they need to collect (Charmaz and Thornberg, 2021). Data tends to be collected through observation or interview and the data analysed, line by line, to better understand what is happening.

Other types of qualitative research

Just like for quantitative research, there are many other types of qualitative methodologies that you may come across and some that might not tell you what specific methodology they have used, other than it was qualitative. Having read this chapter, you should now be able to tell if a piece of research is qualitative or quantitative when you read it by the way it is designed.

Activity 3.10   Critical thinking

Look at the examples below and decide which of the six research designs or methodologies we've described so far might best be used to test/understand/explore these topics. Start by identifying if the statement could be answered by a quantitative- or a qualitative-type question, and then which research design/methodology you could use.

1. Whether cranberry juice is more effective than water in managing the symptoms of a urinary tract infection.
2. An exploration of the experience of mothers caring for a child with a complex health condition.
3. The identification of health risks from vaping in young people.
4. An examination of how nursing associates cope with death and dying in practice.
5. The cultural practices of nurses caring for people with dementia in care homes.
6. The influence of dietary habits on people diagnosed as morbidly obese in relation to those who are not.

As a reminder the six designs we have discussed so far are:

Quantitative designs: RCT, cohort study, case control study
Qualitative methodologies: phenomenology, ethnography, grounded theory

An outline answer is available at the end of the chapter.

Ethics

It is never possible to talk about research without saying something about ethics. As well as ensuring piece of research follows a particular research design, or methodology, it also needs to be carried out *ethically*. Ethical practice is central to healthcare and as a nursing associate you also need to practise ethically at all times.

Working in an ethical way requires you to make *moral* judgements about the care you (and others) provide and, at its most simplistic level, requires you to make judgements about what is morally 'right' and what is morally 'wrong' in everything you do (Cambridge Dictionary, 2023). Every decision you make has the potential to affect others in different ways. We look in greater detail at this, and ethical decision-making in relation to your own practice, in Chapter 6. Here, we consider it in relation to research.

If healthcare is to advance, then research is essential and, unlike in Goffman's time, requires humans (participants/patients) to agree to be part of any research study to enable it to be carried out. Strict guidelines therefore need to be in place to protect those involved. This is particularly true as our understanding of what is ethical changes (and improves) over time – not just because of medical advancements, but also because of our changing and developing understanding of human rights. In fact, there are many examples of unethical practices throughout recent history that we look back at today in horror. We only need look to the Second World War, for example, to find evidence of the atrocities inflicted on prisoners of war during that time. Thousands of men were estimated to have died at the hands of Japanese and German army medics during human experimentation without the men's consent, for example (Harris, 2002). 2022 also saw the 50th anniversary of the Tuskegee Syphilis Study in the US, where public health researchers were known to have intentionally withheld effective treatment for syphilis from African American men, while leading them to believe they were receiving treatment for the condition (Tobin, 2022). More recently, in the UK, there was an outcry when it came to light that hospitals routinely removed and stored hearts of babies and foetuses, following postmortems, for medical experimentation, without the parents' knowledge or consent (Redfern, 2001). While Goffman's undercover study of the asylum may not have harmed lives in the same way as these examples, it still meant that people were being deceived. They believed Goffman was there to do one job, whereas in fact he was there to do another (i.e. to carry out a research study). All of these practices would now be considered unethical.

Although these are mostly extreme examples, and relate to medical ethics, they show the importance of having a clear set of ethical principles for all research that is carried out. The Declaration of Helsinki was first created in 1964 in response to the atrocities that were carried out in the Second World War and to provide a set of principles to guide the ethics of research carried out worldwide. Although this also is medically focused and criticised for focusing too strongly on North American principles (Goodyear et al., 2007), it is used by many countries across the world, including the UK, as a set of guiding principles for what you can and cannot do with regards to research. These principles include:

- ensuring research is of an acceptable standard;
- that it causes no harm and;
- participants in the research will have given their full consent to participate.

(Ellis, 2022)

Following these principles, the NHS Health Research Authority set up a number of *research ethics committees* across the UK to monitor and review the standard of any health-related research *before* it is carried out, requiring researchers to provide a detailed description of each aspect of their proposed study for scrutiny by these panels. Similarly, all universities in the UK will have their own ethics panels and will require any proposed research to be scrutinised by the panel before approval to go ahead with a piece of research is given (or withheld).

It is worth saying, however, that as an undergraduate learner you would *not* carry out a piece of research, although you might be involved in clinical audit. What you will be doing is reading and critiquing research carried out by others and using it to underpin your own practice. Part of the critiquing process is to gauge if the research was carried out ethically.

Carrying out research that isn't valid, is also considered unethical.

Service user (patient) involvement in research

You may recall from Toni's case study that he'd had an accident and was currently using a wheelchair. He also had a grandmother who lived nearby. Below is a transcript of how Toni described what happened when he attempted to visit his grandmother for the first time, using the wheelchair his mother got for him after his accident.

Case study: Toni (part 2)

Mum got me a wheelchair to use while I recovered from my accident and I decided to use it to visit my granny. She lived in a modern house that was designed to be 'accessible' with wide doors and a ramp up the front door. Despite the fact that I visited her all the time, it was only when I arrived in my wheelchair that I noticed, for the first time, that there was a small step up to the ramp, which meant that I couldn't get my wheelchair up it. Because I wasn't allowed to put my foot down, it meant that I couldn't physically reach the doorbell without going up the ramp, but, equally, couldn't go up the ramp in my wheelchair because of the step. I decided instead to try the back door, but to reach it I had to go through the back gate. I quickly discovered that this was too narrow for me to get my wheelchair through. I ended up having to go back to the front door, carefully ease myself out of the wheelchair and hop up the step to reach the doorbell – risking falling over and injuring myself further in the process. It wasn't until I actually tried to get into Granny's house in my wheelchair that I discovered how totally inaccessible her supposedly 'accessible' house was.

Despite the house being built to be accessible to wheelchair users (supposedly), neither the builders, nor Toni himself, while able-bodied, had noticed that a wheelchair user wouldn't actually be able to reach the front door. Having a wheelchair user involved in the planning of the property may have meant that it was better fit for purpose, and oversights such as the example here could have been avoided. Although this may seem an extreme example, it sadly is all too common and shows the importance of involving service users in everything we do; this includes research.

Doing research *with* service users rather than *on* service users is now recognised as essential if the services we design and deliver are truly to meet the needs of those they are intended to serve (Fitzpatrick et al., 2023). Indeed, the main funder of health research (the National Institute for Health Research [NIHR]) in the UK requires service users to be involved in the design of all research that it funds. Have a look at its website at the end of this chapter to see what it says.

The UK also has a set of standards for involving service users in research studies which is worth having a look at. You can find them by searching for UK Standards for Public Involvement.

Activity 3.11 Reflection

Next time you are in your own work area, think about all the equipment you use and whether any of it could have been designed better if a service user had been involved in its design.

As this is based on your own practice, there is no outline answer provided at the end of this chapter.

Chapter summary

Research has its own technical vocabulary, guidelines and standards, and this can mean it can seem intimidating to someone who is unfamiliar with this world. However, learning about the meaning of some of the terms should help you to understand it better; here, we have equipped you with some basic definitions to get you started. We have also shown how research is, in effect, divided into two 'camps': quantitative and qualitative – with each having different (and often opposing) rules that apply to it, as they attempt to understand different things.

Quantitative research, as we have shown, is more interested in testing something and in numbers. Conversely, qualitative research focuses on understanding people's thoughts, habits and behaviours.

There are, however, a number of rules that anyone wanting to carry out health-related research has to abide by and many of these are considered under the umbrella term of 'ethics'. Ensuring research is ethically sound means ensuring that the research does no harm to others: from one extreme of seriously harming or killing someone, to simply wasting their time. Involving service users in the design of research is an important part of this and can ensure that the research is fit for purpose, and the outcomes are meaningful.

In the following chapter you will be using the knowledge you have gained in this chapter in order to help you understand still further the principles of research and continue to 'bust the myths' that can surround it. Developing your skills and confidence in being able to read, understand and critically analyse research will allow you to ensure your practice is informed by evidence from research, improving your evidence-based practice as required in order to be a competent, registered nursing associate.

Activities: Brief outline answers

Activity 3.3 Critical thinking

There might be a number of different reasons for the difference in height.

Sunflowers like a lot of sunshine but prefer to be planted in a sheltered (non-windy) position. They also grow best if they are planted in well-drained soil with added compost and not crowded by other plants.

If there are any differences in how you and your neighbour planted their sunflower, it could affect how tall the sunflowers grow. Equally, it could be that your sunflowers were different varieties, which means that their final full height will inevitably be different.

However, it could just be a random 'chance' that your sunflower ended up being a different height to your neighbour's. Let's say, in this example, that the one difference they found between the two sunflowers was that your neighbour's sunflower was planted in a less sunny position than your own.

Quantitative researchers would look at each of the different variables (the differences between how the two sunflowers were planted and where) to try to identify any differences and drawn their final conclusions regarding sunny/less sunny planting positions. They would then try to work out the likelihood (usually referred to as a *probability*) of their results being correct, or just down to chance. You'll often see this referred to in quantitative studies as the *P value* (p = probability) which is worked out using statistical software. The closer to a zero the *less likely* it is that their results are due to chance. The closer to the number one (often anything greater than 0.05 is considered in this way), the *more likely* it is the results are due to chance. Don't worry too much about how it is calculated: just that you would expect to see a P value in many quantitative papers and that you would normally expect to see a P value of 0.05 or lower. We discuss this again in Chapter 4.

Activity 3.4 Research

The study had three theories that they were testing:

1. that transgender students undertook less physical activity both inside and outside school than non-transgendered students;
2. that transgender youths ate less healthily than non-transgender youths; and
3. that when transgender students felt unsafe at school they were more likely than non-transgender students to behave in ways that were likely to mean they gained weight.

While the researchers of this study believed that transgender students would take less physical activity than non-transgender students, they actually found that this *wasn't* necessarily the case. Although they were less likely to do physical activities *in* the school, they were actually more likely to do it *outside* the school. For Toni, therefore, it may not be that lack of physical activity was the cause of him being overweight.

The researchers did find, however, that transgender youths *may* eat less healthily than non-transgender youths and that this *could* be linked to how safe transgender students felt in school. As Toni felt isolated at school, it might be that there is a connection with how he felt about attending school and his being overweight. However, the researchers did find that youths who were born male were more affected than those (like Toni) who were born female. In addition, you weren't told in the scenario whether Toni was a white Caucasian youth or not; the study by Pistella et al. (2020) found that reports of eating behaviours differed across different ethnic groups. Consequently, we can say that Toni *may* be engaging in unhealthy eating behaviours affected by his experiences in school, but that we can't be absolutely sure that this is the case.

Activity 3.6 Critical thinking

Cohort study data collection. According to the BiB website, they send out regular surveys to participants, collect measurements and biological samples, and routine data from health and medical records.

Activity 3.7 Critical thinking

Quantitative paper: Pistella, J, Ioverno, S, Rodgers, M and Russell, S (2020) The contribution of school safety to weight-related health behaviours for transgender youth. *Journal of Adolescence*, 78: 33–42	Qualitative paper: Medico, D, Sansfaçon, A, Zufferey, A, Galantino, G, Bosom, M and Suerich-Gulick, F (2020) Pathways to gender affirmation in trans-youth: A qualitative and participative study with youth and their parents. *Clinical Child Psychology and Psychiatry*, 25(4): 1002–1014
The initial sample is big (910,885 students) and includes students attending middle and high schools from a specific State in the US	The sample size is small (ten youths and ten parents/caregivers) and 'chosen' because of their allegiance with the organisation 'NGO' and a technique called *snowballing* (where one participant can put the interviewers in touch with other possible participants) is used to get their sample
Uses a structured questionnaire where respondents choose their answers from a set of possible answers provided	Uses interviews which are recorded. The recordings of the interviews are transcribed *verbatum* (in full)
Data are analysed using descriptive statistics (the researchers give you the overall numbers of answers given; they don't 'manipulate' them in any way) and a statistical software package (called StataCorp 2017, version 15) is then used to test how reliable their results are	A data analysis software package MAXQDA is used to order the data, helping the researchers to create a set of themes. Unlike quantitative data packages, qualitative ones don't 'manipulate' data: instead, they are designed to help the researcher organise their data more effectively
Results are presented as a set of figures and tables with some written explanations as to how these were carried out	Results (although referred to as such in this article, many qualitative papers use the term 'findings') are presented as a set of themes which include a series of direct quotes from participants

Activity 3.8 Critical analysis and reflection

Helping Toni is likely to feel like an emotional burden to Sarah. While she might feel that she wants to help, she may feel fearful of saying the wrong thing and may feel helpless at times: but equally that her role is not one that everyone could carry out. She may feel like the 'job' of being a friend to Toni is a 24-hour-a-day responsibility and feel like she is keeping vigil at times, not able to confide in adults at risk of them telling Toni's parents. We aren't told in the case study if Toni is self-harming or feeling suicidal, but, if he is, it is likely that Sarah will need to seek help at some point.

Activity 3.9 Critical thinking and reflection

Ethnographic studies focus on 'taken-for-granted' practices and this article highlights how some heterosexual-biased practices within schools can impact on how non-heterosexual students may feel. Examples given include: toilets and uniforms that may be classified as boy/girl and, in some schools, single-sex classes – all of which can make students who identify as trans feel inferior and marginalised. We don't know anything about Toni's school, but it could be that any of these practices, if they were present, could impact on how Toni felt. The authors of this paper also discuss a 'sexuality and gender diversity support group' at the school where they carried out their research. If there were no similar supportive groups at Toni's school, this could also reinforce his sense of feeling isolated.

Activity 3.10 Critical thinking

Here you were asked to look at the examples below and decide which of the six research designs or methodologies described might *best* be used to test/understand/explore these topics.

Statement: Whether cranberry juice is more effective than water in managing the symptoms of a urinary tract infection.

Answer: Quantitative/RCT

When there is one intervention (in this example it's the cranberry juice) being compared to another intervention (here it is the water) then it will be carried out using an RCT. As we discussed in the chapter, there are different types of RCT (double-blinded or crossover, for example), but they are all considered to be RCTs.

Statement: An exploration of the experience of mothers caring for a child with a complex health condition.

Answer: Qualitative/phenomenology

In this example the researchers are interested in the experiences of mothers. You can see from the statement itself that there is nothing to measure, so the type of research will be qualitative, rather than quantitative. More specifically, where the focus is primarily on experiences then a phenomenological approach might be the most appropriate to use, to better understand what is going on from the mothers' perspectives.

Statement: The identification of health risks from vaping in young people.

Answer: Quantitative/cohort study

In this example you have a quantifiable answer, so would want to use a quantitative approach. However, you couldn't blindly put people into two separate groups and make one group vape and the other not, as it wouldn't be *ethical* to do so. As such, researchers wouldn't be able to use an RCT approach. What they could do is look, prospectively, at a group of young people who do vape and monitor their health over a period of time, in comparison to other young people who don't vape, using a cohort study approach.

Statement: An examination of how nursing associates cope with death and dying in practice.

Answer: Qualitative/grounded theory

This example aims for the researcher to gain a better understanding of an issue. There is nothing measurable here, so the approach would need to be qualitative. An appropriate approach for this topic could be grounded theory, whereby the research aims to understand more about people who share a common experience in order to create a new theory through their deeper understanding.

Statement: The cultural practices of nurses caring for people with dementia in care homes.

Answer: Qualitative/ethnographic

In this example, again, the focus isn't anything that could be measured, so the researcher would use a qualitative approach. When the focus is on a sub-group of people such as this, then an ethnographic approach might be the most appropriate here.

Statement: The influence of dietary habits on people diagnosed as morbidly obese in relation to those who are not.

Answer: Quantitative/case control study

This example was possibly the hardest one of the statements to guess, as it could, in principle, be investigated by either qualitative or quantitative means. However, the best fit for this statement was quantitative research and, most specifically, a case control study. The researcher is comparing two groups; qualitative research doesn't make comparisons, so it has to be quantitative. More specifically, the research is looking at a group of people with a particular condition (the cases) and directly comparing them to those without the condition (the control), making it a case control study.

Annotated further reading

Ellis, P (2022) *Understanding Research for Nursing Students* (5th edition). London: Sage.

This is an introductory text to research and is equally relevant to nursing associates and nursing students. It will be helpful for building, further, your understanding of the principles of research.

Seedhouse, D (2017) *Thoughtful Healthcare: Ethical Awareness and Reflective Practice.* London: Sage.

This is a useful text to help build your understanding of the importance of ethics in relation to research and, more broadly, in relation to your own practice. As such it is equally relevant for both this chapter and Chapter 6 of this book.

Useful websites

www.hra.nhs.uk/

This is the link to the Health Research website and includes the ethical approval checklist that any research carried out within the NHS has to complete.

www.wma.net/policies-post/wma-declaration-of-helsinki-ethical-principles-for-medical-research-involving-human-subjects/

This is a link to the website for the Declaration of Helsinki and identifies what health researchers can and cannot do in the name of research.

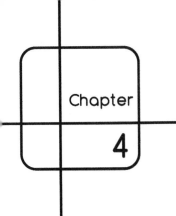

Chapter

4

Critical appraisal of research

Melissa Owens

Chapter aims

After reading this chapter you will be able to:

- appreciate the importance of being able to critique research and its relevance to contemporary practice;
- recognise the difference between good and bad research;
- identify critiquing tools, appropriate to the research being critiqued;
- demonstrate understanding of the key elements of critically appraising the quality of research.

Introduction

As we discussed in Chapter 3, the principles of research can seem overwhelming. Hopefully, by reading this previous chapter, and working through the different exercises, you will now have a better understanding of different research designs and methodologies and feel more confident about what these should look like. In this chapter we build on what you learnt in the last chapter and help to enable you to look at research studies more critically so that you can gauge if they have been carried out well or not. Like other chapters in this book, we provide a list of annotated further readings and websites at the end of the chapter which we think will make useful additional resources. What is new to this chapter, however, is that we introduce some web links to online videos for you to watch. As with understanding the principles of research, we appreciate that the idea of critically appraising research may, at the outset, feel quite scary. But it doesn't need to be. The online video links we include, therefore, have been chosen as they are 'light and entertaining' as well as informative, which we hope will help you, more easily, understand some of the principles we discuss in this chapter and successfully complete all the activities.

Before we start, it might be helpful for you to go back and read Toni's case study, introduced in Chapter 3, as we'll return to his story during some of the discussions in this chapter.

We will continue to use two research papers in this chapter that relate to Toni's case study, and we'd like you to find and read these articles now. If you can't find them, then your librarian should be able to help you.

Activity 4.1   Research

Use your database searching skills to find, and read, the following articles:

1.   Chae, S, Yeo, J, Hwang, J and Kang, H (2021) Effects of school-based 'We Fit' weight control programme in adolescents. *Nursing Open*, 9: 721–732

and

2.   Mikovits, J (2022) I don't feel like I'm a person: Nursing knowledge of transgender care through the lens of transgender people. *Journal of Advanced Nursing*, 78: 3012–3024

   There is no outline answer to this activity at the end of the chapter.

Thinking critically about research

In Chapter 3 we also told you that it was beyond the realms of that chapter to go into any great detail about the different research designs and methodologies and advised you to find a research book that you found easy to read. We also suggested one that you might find helpful in the annotated reading section. You will find it helpful to have this book to hand for this chapter too. As a reminder the reference for this book is here:

Ellis, P (2022) *Understanding Research for Nursing Students* (5th edition). London: Sage.

Now let's start to think about how we critically appraise research by having a go at the following activity. You might not see the relevance to start with, but, hopefully, thinking about the answers will help you to appreciate that you probably already have some critiquing skills before you even start looking at any research papers.

Activity 4.2   Critical thinking

We are constantly bombarded with advertisements, everywhere we look. However, have you ever thought about the facts behind the headlines they try to sell us? Below, we've written three of our own headlines for some fictitious products. Have a look at them and write down anything you consider might be wrong with the statements and what else you would need to know before deciding if the claims are true or not.

- 80 per cent of women believe they'd lose weight using our product
- There's no other dog food my dog prefers more
- Our hairspray guarantees to hold your hair in place all day* additional products may be required

An outline answer is available at the end of the chapter.

How many of the answers at the end of the chapter did you think of? This wasn't a definitive list and you may have thought of others. This exercise will hopefully have shown you that you need to have an understanding of the facts behind the headlines, and will help you with the critiquing of research papers that we will get you to do later in this chapter. If an advertiser makes a statement such as: '80 per cent of women believe they'd lose weight using our product', you would want to know what questions were asked of respondents in order for the researchers to draw this conclusion (even if they were appropriate questions to ask, which they weren't). How do you know, for example, that the questions were asked in an unbiased way that didn't sway the people they surveyed to give a particular answer?

Activity 4.3   Critical thinking

Below is a link to a YouTube video. Copy the link into a web browser and watch the video entitled 'For and Against National Service'. The clip is from a comedy series shown in the UK in the 1980s called *Yes, Prime Minister*. Although the clip is now dated, and is fictitious, the principles that they discussed still hold relevance today. In this three-and-a-half-minute clip, they discuss how opinion polls can be swayed to give totally opposing responses, depending on the questions that are asked.

Have a look at the clip now: www.youtube.com/watch?v=ahgjEjJkZks

There is no outline answer at the end of the chapter.

Although the clip is from a fictitious comedy drama, the principles equally apply to real-life research you will read today. Certainly, they often apply to the advertisements that we are bombarded with on the television and online media. All research, therefore, needs to be transparent and open for critical appraisal so that others can judge for themselves how robust the research actually was.

Activity 4.4   Critical thinking

Now watch this next video clip called '10 heads in a row' by Derren Brown showing how he is able to toss a coin and get it to come up 'heads' ten times in a row. He assures us, at the start of the clip, that he did this under controlled conditions with multiple cameras to ensure there was no trickery involved. Copy the link into a web browser and watch the video now and try to work out how he did, genuinely, manage to toss a coin and it come up ten heads in a row:

www.youtube.com/watch?v=XzYLHOX50Bc

Once you've thought of your answer, have a look at the next video clip to see how he does it. The discussion about this experiment starts a minute and ten seconds into the clip:

www.youtube.com/watch?v=n1SJ-Tn3bcQ

There is no outline answer at the end of the chapter for this activity.

Had you worked out how he did it correctly? It seems obvious once you know: but that's because you now have the whole picture: unlike when you watched the first one. Hopefully, this helps you understand further why it's so important to see the whole picture and how researchers got to the conclusions that they drew.

Throwing ten heads in a row *is* possible, as you've just seen. However, the likelihood (or the *probability*, which is the term generally used in research) is very small. When carrying out their own research, researchers should tell you the probability (the *p* value) of their own results having happened by chance; the smaller the *p* value, the more we can rely on their results. Normally, anything less than 0.05 is considered 'okay'; anything less than 0.02 is good.

Now let's translate what you now know into a statement that relates to healthcare research.

Although there might be some rare exceptions (like Wakefield's (1998) research that we mentioned in previous chapters) (Rao and Andrade, 2011), research that you see published in journals shouldn't, intentionally, set out to deceive you. However, that still doesn't mean that the research has necessarily been carried out well.

Activity 4.5   Critical thinking

Have a read of the following statement and write down a list of things you might need to know/consider before you believe it to be true or not. The statement isn't based on any specific research per se, so there is no 'right' or 'wrong' answer, but is meant to reflect something you might typically hear in the media, your place of work, your college or university.

'Hospital waiting times have increased by 50 per cent in the past five years'

Some suggestions as to what you might identify are included at the end of this chapter.

Again, this activity was to get you thinking about the facts behind the headlines that you might hear and not just to accept what you are told without question. It was also to help to continue to build your confidence and appreciation further, to reassure you that you probably know something about critiquing research, even if you didn't realise it: because again, in essence, that was what you were being asked to do in this activity.

Transparency is at the heart of all good-quality research and having all the information available is paramount in ensuring it can be judged by others so that we can believe their results. Consider, for example, the next time you collect a prescription for medication from your doctor. You take it in the belief that it has been researched thoroughly and is safe to take. But how would you feel if there was a 'cloak and dagger' around the research evidence behind the medicine? If the research wasn't available to be scrutinised? In fact, there is a lot of criticism around what is known as *publication bias*, with researchers only publishing the results of studies they *want* you to see, where the results were what they *expected* them to be. Equally, however, this is criticism of publishers only publishing the results of research where the findings are interesting. This means that some research never gets read and that, therefore, we only have part of the total picture: the ten coins being tossed in a row.

Activity 4.6   Critical thinking

Copy the following link into your web browser and watch the following video called: 'Ben Goldacre: Battling Bad Science'. It is a Ted Talk that is available via YouTube. It is a little dated now (it was recorded in 2011), but still relevant today; we feel it will be really helpful in enabling you to understand the principles we discuss in this chapter and the critiquing activities that we go on to discuss shortly.

www.youtube.com/watch?v=h4MhbkWJzKk

There is no outline answer for this activity at the end of this chapter.

Goldacre is a champion advocating for all research data, and research studies themselves, to be published, whatever the results, but also openly challenges any headline where the data is either unavailable or questionable. We suggest two of his books in the Further reading section at the end of this chapter.

Another criticism made about research papers is that, even when they are published, they are not readily available to all. How easily did you find the two research papers we asked you to find at the start of this chapter? Did you find them more easily than the ones we asked you to find in the previous chapter? If you have answered 'yes' to this second question, the reason is probably because both of these papers are available through what is called *open access*, whereas only one of the papers we asked you to find in the previous chapter was. You can usually tell if a paper is open access because it has a picture of a little unlocked padlock in the top right-hand corner of the article; normally it will state this when you do a database search through your organisation, college, or university library. We discussed further steps to find papers in the previous chapter.

Critiquing research

For your studies and your work, you will need to develop your critiquing skills so that you can critique research in a systematic way. Hopefully, from having completed the exercises above, you will appreciate that you can't simply rely on reading the final conclusion to a piece of research: you need to look at *how* the conclusion was reached. To do that, you will need some understanding of the *principles* behind different pieces of research that we discussed in the previous chapter. In addition, you will need a tool or a checklist to help you identify different parts of a research paper to examine in greater detail. Thankfully, there are a number of critiquing tools that are readily available to help you do this in a systematic way so let's have a look at some of them now.

The CASP (Critical Appraisal Skills Programme) is a useful place to start when looking for a critiquing tool as the website provides a series of different tools for different types of research. They are also provided in a format that allows the user to populate the checklist electronically, and are reviewed and updated regularly. There is also a short glossary of some useful terms provided that you might find in the research articles you read (https://casp-uk.net/glossary/) and the tools have a clear focus on the results and their relevance for clinical practice.

The first research paper that we asked you to read in the previous chapter was by Pistella et al. (2020); it was a quantitative study that didn't align itself to any particular research design. Similarly, the two articles we asked you to find at the start of this chapter don't either. Although CASP provides a generic CASP tool for qualitative research, it doesn't provide one for quantitative research; therefore, finding a CASP tool to use for both the Pistella et al. (2020) and the Chae et al. (2021) papers to help you critique them would be difficult. In examples such as this, it's probably more helpful to use a generic tool for quantitative research. There are many that are available and most have been in use for a number of years. However, we suggest one for quantitative research and a similar one for qualitative research here which break down the critiquing process into reasonable bite-sized, not-too-technical chunks.

Activity 4.7   Critical thinking

Use your database searching skills to find, and read, the following articles:

1. Coughlan, M, Cronin, P and Ryan, F (2007) Step-by-step guide to critiquing research. Part 1: quantitative research. *British Journal of Nursing*, 16(11): 658–663.
2. Ryan, F, Coughlan, M and Cronin, P (2007) Step-by-step guide to critiquing research. Part 2: qualitative research. *British Journal of Nursing*, 16(12): 738–744.

We will use these two papers as a focus for the remainder of the chapter.

Look at the research questions in Table 4.1 for each of these papers. The first provides a checklist-type summary of the different questions to ask when critiquing either a quantitative (paper 1) or qualitative (paper 2) paper.

What are the similarities and differences between the questions for the two different types of research?
There is an outline answer at the end of this chapter.

You will have seen, when you read these papers, that the authors break their questions down into two broad sections: aspects of the research that relate to the *believability* of the research (how it's written, who wrote it, the title and the abstract) and those aspects of the research that relate to how well the research was carried out (the remainder of the research process). You will also have seen that the questions in the section relating to believability of the research are identical for both. Within the next section, some of the questions are the same and some differ. However, even if the question is the same, such as those relating to *sample*, you will notice that the explanations of what it means might differ, whereas others – such as *ethical considerations* – remain the same. As we discussed in the previous chapter, quantitative and qualitative research principles are very different and it's important not to try to apply the 'rules' of quantitative research to qualitative and vice versa. To help you with this, we are going to look at critiquing both types of research side by side.

So where should you begin when you are trying to critique a research paper? In the previous chapter we told you not to worry about any terms you didn't understand at the time in the research papers we asked you to read. However, now you are starting to think about critiquing, you will need to understand them; making a note of any terms you don't understand, is a good place to start.

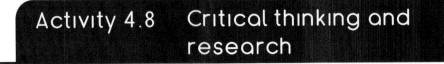

Activity 4.8 Critical thinking and research

At the start of this chapter, we asked you to find two research papers: Chae et al. (2021) and Mikovits (2022).

1. Read these papers again and make a note of any terms you don't understand; keep these as your own glossary.
2. Now we want you to find the meaning for all the terms that you don't understand; but, before you do, read the following quote and the remainder of the guidance provided in this activity box. Have a read of what one of our authors said when they were first learning something new.

> When I first started studying, I was asked to critique the writing style of a research article. This included an in-depth analysis of the grammar that they'd used. However, my understanding of English grammar was pretty poor. When I learnt grammar at school, we weren't explicitly taught the principles, but were just sort of expected to absorb them. I had conscientiously brought all the reading books on the reading list for the module, but when I opened them I didn't understand a word! I therefore took myself out shopping and ended up buying a book on grammar for 11-year-olds. It was the best thing I ever did. I was able to learn the meaning of basic grammar principles and gradually work my way up until I could understand the books that were on the reading list.
> *Published with permission*

Although we don't expect you to need a book aimed at 11-year-olds, the same principle does apply: find something that helps you make sense of the research terms that you don't understand, but don't feel that it needs to be a 'high-brow' textbook. In fact, it doesn't even necessarily need to be a book. YouTube has lots of videos on different aspects of research and, although you shouldn't cite it in your essays, Wikipedia can also be useful as a starting point (but no more than that) to help you understand a basic principle. A Google search may also be all you need. These suggestions may feel as if they go against the grain of what we (and your lecturers) have been teaching you so far, but remember you are only using these as building blocks to help you gain some understanding and confidence of terms you might not understand.

There is no outline answer at the end of the chapter for this activity.

Once you have some confidence and understand the general principles of the terms used in these research papers, you might want to build up your understanding a bit further by having a look at the CASP glossary we mentioned earlier: https://casp-uk.net/glossary/, as well the research book by Ellis (2022) that we recommended to you in the previous chapter and earlier on in this one. You might also want to find additional research texts that explain the general research terms and are written in a way that makes sense to you.

Activity 4.9 Critical thinking and research

Return to the two articles on critiquing research by Coughlan et al. (2007) and Ryan et al. (2007) that we asked you to read earlier. Look at the first set of questions on elements influencing believability of the research and have a go at critiquing the Chae et al. (2021) and Mikovits (2022) papers.

Are there any more questions you think you would want to ask in this section?

You will probably find that you have to read the articles more than once to get a sense of them and that's absolutely as we would expect.

There is an outline answer at the end of this chapter.

From doing this activity you will, hopefully, appreciate that there is no *absolute* right or wrong answer to every question; it is based on your judgement, but that judgement needs to be founded in evidence. How good is your grammar, for example, in order to be able to judge that of the authors? This is where your textbooks will be essential. You may find, like in the example from one of our authors above, that you need to start out with something really basic, but as your understanding and confidence grow you will find that you will be able to read and understand more complex texts that will enable you to look at research papers in more depth.

Activity 4.10 Critical thinking and research

Now that you've had a go at using the first set of questions from the Coughlan et al.'s (2007) and Ryan et al.'s (2007) critiquing tools, have a go at the second section: elements influencing the *robustness* of the research. You may think this section is harder than the first, but it shouldn't be as you will have the knowledge you gained from the previous chapter, the activities you've already completed in this chapter and your research text books to help you.

There is an outline answer at the end of this chapter.

How did you find this activity? Some of the terminology can seem challenging, so do persevere with looking up, and reading around, the more complex terms to help you understand them better. Once you've felt you have answered all the questions have a go at this one, final, activity of the chapter.

Activity 4.11   Critical thinking

Having critiqued both papers for the exercise above, now decide the following:

- how well do you think each piece of research was carried out?
- do you think one was carried out better than the other?
- returning to the case study of Toni, was there anything in either study that might help you better understand Toni's healthcare needs?

There is an outline answer at the end of this chapter.

Chapter summary

Critiquing research can feel like a difficult skill to learn. However, hopefully by introducing you to a set of step-by-step skills, you will now feel more confident in how to do it. Remember that you don't need to start with a text book or article that feels so complicated that you don't understand it. Find something that works for you and gradually build up to more complex texts bit by bit. By doing this you should be able to build up both your confidence and your skills to enable you to critique research and consider its relevance to your own practice.

Activities: Brief outline answers

Activity 4.2 Critical thinking

In this activity we asked you to think about what else you might need to know in order to establish the 'truth' behind the headlines of three different advertisements that we had invented. Here are some of the things that you might have included in your answers.

80 per cent of women believe they'd lose weight using our product

Beware whenever you see a percentage without the actual numbers presented alongside it. If there were only five people asked, for example, 80 per cent would have a very different meaning to if it was 80 per cent of 1000.

Have you ever used a weight-losing product? If you have, you probably did so because you wanted to lose weight and therefore *believed* that the product would help you achieve that goal. It's possible that four out of five perhaps, or 800 out of 1000 – i.e. 80 per cent of women – would believe the same. This headline, therefore, doesn't actually tell you what you really want to know, which is how likely it is to work.

We also don't know what question the women were asked before they gave their answer. How do we know the question didn't lead them to answer one way over another?

There's no other dog food my dog prefers more

If you look at this statement carefully you will see that the statement isn't actually saying that the dog prefers one dog food over another, just that there isn't another it prefers more. In other words, the product could be just as good (or as bad) as any other.

This statement also brings into question sample sizes. Can we really believe something is good, or that it works, because one dog believes it to be the case? Different dogs may have different preferences: or have been fed just one product since they were a puppy, meaning that they have acquired a taste for it and wouldn't want another. Consider, also, how would you feel about taking a drug that had been trialled on just one person – who may or may not have similar characteristics (such as age, sex, health status) – as yourself? You wouldn't want to. As we discussed in the previous chapter when looking at RCTs, you would want the product to be tested on a sample that was representative of the (in this example dog) population as a whole.

You would also want to know what other products were used in the comparison. How many were there (again, did they truly represent the different products that were available)?

Our hairspray guarantees to hold your hair in place all day*

*additional products may be required

In this example the claim is that a product will 'guarantee' something; in actual fact, it isn't guaranteeing it at all because it's saying you might need to use other products as well in order to hold your hair in place. As we discussed in the previous chapter when looking at RCTs, the researcher needs to be sure, conclusively, that the results they get are due to the 'thing' being tested and not anything else.

Again, in this sample we don't know what the sample looks like. How many people was it tested on and what hair types did they have? Does it work better for one hair type over another? It also doesn't say what weather conditions it was tested in. Does this depend if you go outside or not? If it rains or not? Or if the wind is blowing?

Activity 4.5 Critical thinking

It's important that you don't just accept *carte blanche* what you read, or hear, in the media or from your colleagues. The first thing you should ask is: does it sound realistic? Whatever your answer, then ask yourself 'Why?' Here are a few things to consider in relation to the statements from this activity.

Hospital waiting times have increased by 50 per cent in the past five years

With everything we hear in the news, you might well think this is true, but you might also want to consider what might have impacted on healthcare delivery over this period. For example:

- strikes by nurses and doctors;
- ongoing shortages of nurses and doctors;
- the ongoing impact of COVID-19 and treatments being put 'on hold' during the COVID-19 years;
- the crisis within the social care sector causing discharge delays for patients.

It's also important to look at how an 'increase in waiting times' is measured. For example, does it include planned treatments and outpatient appointments or is it just measuring those turning up at Accident and Emergency departments? You may not have thought about planned treatments when you first looked at this statement, so it's also worth considering exactly which waiting times are included in this figure. For a closer look at what is officially measured details are provided on the NHS England website: www.england.nhs.uk/statistics/

You should also be aware of anything that has a percentage in it rather than actual figures. If you have a room with one person in it and another person enters, you could, in theory, say that the number of people in the room has increased by 100 per cent! Although that is an extreme example, our brains are able to process real numbers better than percentages, and it does show how meaningless a percentage can be unless given alongside the actual figures.

Activity 4.7 Critical thinking

The authors divide their checklists into two sections, the first being elements influencing the *believability* of the research and the second being elements influencing the *robustness* of the research. The questions in the first section are the same in both checklists, but differ, to some degree, in the second. Table 4.1 highlights, in bold, those elements that are the same in both checklists.

Table 4.1

Paper 1: checklist for quantitative research (Coughlan et al., 2007)	Paper 2: checklist for qualitative research (Ryan et al., 2007)
Writing style	**Writing style**
Author	**Author**
Report title	**Report title**
Abstract	**Abstract**
Purpose/research problem	Statement of phenomenon of interest
Logical consistency	**Purpose**/significance of the study
Literature review	**Literature review**
Theoretical framework	**Theoretical framework**
Aims/objectives/research question/hypothesis	Method and philosophical underpinnings
Sample	**Sample**
Ethical considerations	**Ethical considerations**
Operational definitions	Data collection/**data analysis**
Methodology	Rigour
Data analysis/results	Findings/discussion
Discussion	Conclusions/implications/recommendations
References	**References**

Activity 4.9 Critical thinking and research

Table 4.2

Paper 1 (Chae et al., 2021)	Paper 2 (Mikovits, 2022)
Writing style	
This paper follows a logical format, uses grammar appropriately, avoids jargon and is well organised.	This paper follows a logical format, uses grammar appropriately, with minor errors, avoids jargon and is well organised. However, it is common to write qualitative research in the first person; in this paper the author refers to themselves as 'the researcher' throughout.
The authors of this paper appear to have English as their second language and some flexibility can be given for this. However, it isn't needed on this occasion.	The author of this paper appears to have English as a second language and some flexibility can be given for this.
Author	
There are four authors given for this paper and their affiliated institutions are all listed, with an email address provided for the correspondent author. They all appear to work in nursing-related fields, although the paper doesn't spell out if the authors are nurses or not. No qualifications are provided.	There is just the one author for this paper, who is a PhD student at the time of writing. They provide the name of their affiliated institution as well as their email address.
Report title	
The title is clear, accurate and unambiguous.	The title is clear, accurate and unambiguous.
Abstract	
The abstract offers a clear overview of the study, including the different stages of the research process.	The abstract offers a clear overview of the study, including the different stages of the research process.

We also asked you to consider if there were any other questions that you might want to ask here. Having watched the YouTube video by Ben Goldacre, you might also have wanted to know if the author(s) had any conflicting interests – for example, being funded by a drug company. Chae et al. (2021) do declare funding for their research from the National Research Foundation of Korea and 'overseas training expenses' from Seoul National University, neither of which appear to be private funders who could profit from the results of the study.

Activity 4.10 Critical thinking and research

Table 4.3

Paper 1 (Chae et al., 2021)	Paper 2 (Mikovits, 2022)
Purpose/research problem	**Statement of the phenomenon of interest**
This is clearly stated as being to examine 'the effects of a 12-week school-based *"We Fit"* weight control problem'.	This is clearly stated and focuses on people who identify as transgender, their experiences of healthcare delivery, interactions with

registered nurses and how this might influence their seeking future healthcare. The author argues that most research focuses on the LGBTQ community as a whole and healthcare as a whole, rather than specifically with registered nurses. The phenomenon of interest is consistent with the study aims.

Logical consistency

Yes. These are clearly labelled under the sub-headings used.

Purpose/significance of the study

The purpose of the study is clearly stated as being: 'to discover and understand the perceptions of healthcare delivery for transgender people who have had interactions with nurses while receiving care' and 'to identify if these perceptions of nursing knowledge have an influence on transgender individuals seeking future healthcare' (p. 3012).

Two aims are identified and, although the researcher states he also had a research question, this isn't included.

Literature review

The literature review is presented under the heading 'background'. It cites a number of other studies, some going back to 2006 but others more recent to when this study was carried out.

It is logically organised and cites a number of research studies, but it is not clear how the papers cited were selected and whether the process used was systematic or not.

The review confirms an association of healthy eating and exercise with positive mental health and argues that peer support is a good way to encourage this. However, although the authors state that adolescents may have misperceptions of their body weight, this isn't explored further. Neither is the potentially negative impact of peer support/potential pressure on exercising in front of others if/when conscious of body shape and size. However, the role that peer support can play is recognised.

The researchers cite a previous study confirming the effectiveness of combining diet, exercise and behavioural therapy to be effective. However, they confirm that using *exergaming* (exercise using video games) has not previously been researched, thereby confirming the uniqueness of their own study.

There is a literature review provided with a clear process as to how papers met/did not meet inclusion criteria and how many were included. However, there is limited discussion as to the content of these papers themselves.

Theoretical framework

The authors state they used a non-equivalent control group alongside a non-synchronised pre-test–post-test design. However, this means that the programme is measured against 'no intervention' rather than the 'next-best', or a similar intervention, even though they identify these in their literature review.

The research terms used aren't explained.

There is a brief explanation of the transtheoretical model which is used to divide students into one of three intervention groups, based on weight control and attitude, which appeared appropriate.

Aims/objectives/research question/hypothesis

The aim is stated in the abstract and again in the paper itself. It relates back to the literature review (background) in terms of weight control and physical activity, but not in relation to unhealthy eating. There is no, actual, research question. Neither is there a hypothesis for this research. There are no obectives stated.

The focus of the research does relate to the focus of the literature review.

The author uses a qualitative, interpretive, descriptive approach, which is appropriate for the design of the study. However, only a limited description of this is provided.

A constant-comparative analytical approach was used, which is appropriate for the research. However, only a limited description is provided.

The concept of *bracketing* is also applied and, again, is appropriate for this type of research, but with little description provided.

Method and philosophical underpinnings

The paper starts by stating a belief that people from LGBTQ communities face stigma, harassment and discrimination and this can lead to them facing barriers and inequitable access to healthcare.

The author also starts with the premise that this same community is likely to face greater health issues in comparison to the general population, including sexually transmitted diseases, mental health issues and suicide risk.

Evidence is provided to support these claims, which appears appropriate.

The author uses in-depth, virtual interviews to gather data; this method is explained in detail.

Sample

The study involved 10th and 11th grade students, aged 15 to 17 years of age, from one private high school in Seoul. The participants had to be able to understand Korean, self-report as healthy and consent, along with their parents, to their participating in the study. Being from one school and in Korea limits the generalisability of this study.

Participants were recruited using a convenience sample and G-Power was used to ascertain the sample size required for the study, which was met.

Simple cluster sampling was used, with 127 students from five classes included and randomly divided into two groups (two classes of 60 in the intervention and three classes of 67 in the control group). Eighteen students

A sampling method of *purposive sampling* was used for the study. Inclusion/exclusion criteria were provided and those included clearly reflected the aims of the study, rendering the participants appropriate for informing the research.

Purposive sampling is an appropriate sampling method for qualitative research and a rationale for its use is justified by the author. However, although the author justifies the number of participants used in the study as ten, they were each only interviewed once and it was, therefore, difficult to see how saturation could be reached.

dropped out, leaving 50 in the intervention group and 59 in the control group.

Of the 18 students that dropped out of the programme; 11 of these cases were due to poor compliance with wearing the activity tracker. This meant their data would be missing from the final results, which would then be skewed.

Ethical considerations

The authors obtained ethical approval from the Institutional Review Board of the first author's university and the reference number for this is provided.

The authors argue, in the literature review section, that the research is unique. It is unethical to carry-out research that isn't necessary and a waste of participants' time. Therefore, they justify the ethicality of the research in terms of uniqueness here.

Ethical approval was sought from both the participants and, because of their age, their parents, although we are not shown copies of the consent forms used.

The authors approached the students personally, rather than via a third party, which could make them feel coerced. However, students had to return consent forms from their parents, meaning that they would have a 'cooling off period', should they decide not to take part.

Operational definitions

There is no specific pilot study carried out. However, qualitative focus groups are used to help develop the programme with the students themselves, alongside a literature review, identifying weight control behaviours with body mass indexes in adolescents and consulting different professionals including the school principal, physical education teachers, school nurse and school dietician.

The overall goal is to establish effectiveness of the programme in terms of anthropometric and physiological factors as well as programme satisfaction. The lack of specific objectives means that how these will be measured isn't clear at the outset.

The author obtained ethical approval from the Institutional Review Board from the institution where he was undertaking his research.

The author argues, in the introduction, how limited research has been carried out with people who are transgender specifically in relation to their interactions with registered nurses and healthcare. Therefore, they justify the ethicality of the research in terms of uniqueness here.

A mental health resource sheet was given to participants for use if needed.

Participation was voluntary and with adults who were able to give their own consent.

Participants' names were anonymised to ensure their identity was protected. All were allowed to choose their own pseudonyms.

All interviews were carried out virtually.

Data were stored on a password-protected computer.

Data collection/data analysis

The author uses in-depth interviews with the ten participants to collect their data. The length of interviews is recorded and interview questions provided.

A constant-comparative method for data analysis is used and described within the paper. This is an appropriate method for this type of research. The interviews took place via Zoom and were recorded and then transcribed. These transcripts are used as part of the data analysis process.

The sample size is justified in relation to achieving saturation, but no clarification is provided as to how saturation is achieved.

Methodology

The research design is clearly identified.

The 12-week programme used a non-equivalent control group, with a non-synchronised pre-test–post-test design. However, as discussed above, the results would have been more meaningful if the programme was tested against the 'next-best' or an equivalent healthy-weight programme.

Focus groups were carried out to explore students' weight control needs and the proposed programme was reviewed, and feedback given, by the school health professionals (identified above).

All adolescents were encouraged to take part, irrespective of weight.

Participation involved: exergaming (playing activity-type video games), keeping a diet diary, individual counselling via text messaging, face-to-face health education provided by the school nurse alongside small-group discussions via text messages. However, by including a number of different elements, it isn't possible to establish whether it is one individual element, or a combination of elements, in the programme that made it effective.

Sociodemographic variables were self-reported via questionnaire, but the honesty of this self-recording wasn't tested.

Physioloical characteristics were measured against the 'INBODY J10', criteria although we are not given details of the content of this.

Blood tests were taken to measure lipids, high-density lipoprotein cholesterol, low-density lipoprotein cholesterol, total cholesterol, triglyceride and glucose levels.

Physical activity was measured by daily step counts, using a Fitbit Zip, alongside daily sitting time. An eight-day baseline was taken with a 12-week follow-up. However, sitting time was measured by asking students to record how many hours they sat for each day and we are not told how this was tested to ensure how honesty or accuracy was monitored in the recording.

Programme satisfaction was measured via a questionnaire issued to the intervention group, five weeks after the programme was completed, using five, open-ended questions, which are included in the article. However, recall could affect responses.

Rigour

The author discusses rigour in a number of ways under the sub-heading 'Validity and reliability/rigour' (p. 3016).

The author describes how they used *interpretative description* as a design to ensure validity and reliability (p. 3012). They describe how they used bracketing, and an interpretative approach, in an attempt to ensure the findings represented the voices of the participants, rather than their own. However, there is only a limited discussion as to how this was achieved.

The author describes how they kept field notes and documented their analytical thinking. They also kept an audit trail to demonstrate how they analysed their data set. This was only carried out by themselves, however, with no second reviewer used to confirm their findings.

Data analysis/results

Statistical analysis is carried out using STATA V14.0.

The Kolmogorov–Smirnov test was used to assess normality of variables.

Descriptive parameters were used to describe the distribution of demographic data.

Categorical variables were tested using the chi-square and Mann-Whiney U tests.

Students complete a 'programme satisfaction' questionnaire at the end of the programme. Forty-three out of 59 (73%) of the students reported positive changes to their eating habits, but we are not told if this is significant. Thirty-one (53%) state they will try to eat more healthily in the future, but, again, we are not told if this is significant. Neither does it measure actual behaviour. We are not told what measures are taken to ensure the students answer the questions honestly and don't simply write what they believe the researchers want to hear. In addition, recall could also affect responses.

The TREND reporting guidelines are used, but we aren't provided with a copy of these.

The researchers also report changes to cholesterol levels, waist circumferences and muscle mass. However, as this was not followed up later, we do not know if these changes were maintained. In addition, the programme included students who did not need to alter their weight and these are not reported separately.

Results for those in the control group are tested at a different time of year to the intervention group, meaning they were tested during different seasons which could impact on the results gathered.

The *P value* is cited as <0.05, which means the results can be considered statistically significant.

Discussion

The limitations of the study are not specifically linked back to the literature review.

Many limitations of the study are identified, including those mentioned above. However, the validity of using a control group that had no intervention was not discussed.

Findings/discussion

The findings are presented as a set of themes, with some direct quotes provided to support these. This is an appropriate way to present findings for qualitative research.

Conclusions/implications/recommendations

The importance and implications of the findings are identified and recommendations for how the findings can be developed are provided. However, more time is spent discussing current healthcare access issues than future access concerns.

References

All references cited in the article are included in the reference list. Some references, however, are more than ten years old, which should be the date limit for references used.

All references cited in the article are included in the reference list. Two references, however, are only given as abbreviations in the body of the article, leaving the reader to work out to which references, in the reference list, they referred.

Overall, references used were current to the publication date and relevant to the study.

Activity 4.11 Critical thinking

How well do you think each piece of research was carried out?

Paper 1 (Chae et al., 2021) uses a quantitative design to measure the effectiveness of a specific health-intervention programme on adolescents. However, the programme is made up of a variety of separate elements and it isn't possible, therefore, to ascertain whether any single element was effective or not. It also compares the programme to 'no intervention' rather than a different type of intervention. Therefore, we have nothing against which to judge the effectiveness, so don't know if it is any better or worse than other interventions.

Paper 2 (Mikovits, 2022) uses a qualitative methodology to explore the experiences of accessing healthcare for adults identifying as transgender, their interactions with registered nurses and if this may impact on future access expectations. Overall, the research is carried out robustly, although the number of participants used in the study is small and may impact on the overall findings.

Do you think one was carried out better than the other?

We felt that paper 2 was carried out better than paper 1, due to the reasons given above.

Was there anything in either study that might help you better understand Toni's healthcare needs?

While paper 1 focused on adolescents, and on managing weight, the students were from a different culture, which could impact on the transferability of the study to people in the UK. In addition, Toni identifies as transgender which may impact on his motivation to join in a programme within his school itself. In addition, the peer support the authors cite as positive could have been considered a negative element to Toni.

Paper 2 focuses specifically on people who are transgender, but the participants are adults, rather than adolescents. However, concerns regarding *dead naming* and using incorrect pronouns may equally be experienced by Toni. Although the study is carried out in the US, the culture of America is more similar to the UK than that of Korea, which should mean that this research is more readily transferable. Concerns regarding attitudes of nurses could help nursing associates in the UK be more aware of the language they use, and how they interact with patients who identify as transgender.

Annotated further reading

Goldacre, B (2010) *Bad Science*. London: Fourth Estate.

The author describes his book as 'pop science'. It is written in an easy-to-follow way. Chapter 8 focuses specifically on statistical errors relating to healthcare, so if you only want to read one chapter then this is the chapter to read.

Goldacre, B (2015) *I Think You'll Find it's a Bit More Complicated Than That.* London: Fourth Estate.

This book contains a series of real-life research studies that the author looks at in more detail and then pulls apart. This is a good text to read to help build your confidence in how many errors research studies can contain.

Useful websites

www.bbc.co.uk/programmes/b006qshd

This is a link to a Radio 4 programme called More or Less which looks at the facts behind the statistics we hear in the media. There are 100s of episodes to listen to and many of them include those relating to health and social care.

https://casp-uk.net/casp-tools-checklists/

CASP: a number of free tools checklists to help you perform critical appraisals.

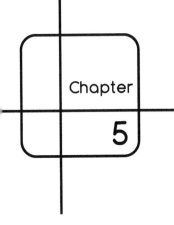

Health inequalities, evidence-based practice and the nursing associate

Hannah Smith

NMC STANDARDS OF PROFICIENCY FOR NURSING ASSOCIATES

This chapter will address the following platforms and proficiencies:

Platform 1: Being an accountable professional

1.4   demonstrate an understanding of, and the ability to, challenge or report discriminatory behaviour

1.11   provide, promote, and where appropriate advocate for, non-discriminatory, person-centred, and sensitive care at all times. Reflect on people's values and beliefs, diverse backgrounds, cultural characteristics, language requirements, needs and preferences, taking account of any need for adjustments

1.15   take responsibility for continuous self-reflection, seeking and responding to support and feedback to develop professional knowledge and skills

1.17   safely demonstrate evidence-based practice in all skills and procedures stated in Annexes A and B

Platform 2: Promoting health and preventing ill health

2.3   describe the principles of epidemiology, demography, and genomics and how these may influence health and wellbeing outcomes

2.4   understand the factors that may lead to inequalities in health outcomes

Platform 3: Provide and monitor care

3.10   demonstrate the knowledge, skills and ability to act as required to meet people's needs related to mobility, hygiene, oral care, wound care and skin integrity

3.11   demonstrate the ability to recognise when a person's condition has improved or deteriorated by undertaking health monitoring. Interpret, promptly respond, share findings, and escalate as needed

3.20   understand and apply the principles and processes for making reasonable adjustments

Platform 6: Contributing to integrated care

6.2   understand and explore the challenges of providing safe nursing care for people with complex co-morbidities and complex care needs

6.5   identify when people need help to facilitate equitable access to care, support and escalate concerns appropriately

> # Chapter aims
>
> After reading this chapter you will be able to:
>
> - understand what is meant by health inequalities in Britain today;
> - examine how health inequalities impact the patients in your care;
> - develop an awareness of your role as a nursing associate in applying evidence-based practice in reducing health inequalities.

Introduction

Of all the forms of inequality, injustice in healthcare is the most shocking and inhumane.

Dr Martin Luther King Jr

So far in this book we have offered you an overview of the history and relevance of evidence-based practice (EBP) (Chapter 1) and provided you with the tools to understand, seek out and critique research in order to help you use it in your own practice (Chapters 2, 3 and 4). The remainder of this book will look at helping you understand how it is applied within differing contexts. The first of these remaining chapters looks at health inequalities: what they are and their significance in relation to evidence-based practice, both in the context of healthcare and your own practice as a nursing associate. Using the activities within this chapter, you will be supported to think about the knowledge, skills and behaviours you have acquired in your career in healthcare to date, considering the evidence-base behind these, but (importantly in the context of this chapter) to do so alongside your personal beliefs and attitudes. You will be guided to consider how protected characteristics, as outlined in the Equality Act (EHRC, 2010), and the social determinants of health as outlined by the World Health Organization (WHO, n.d.) can impact an individual, and what evidenced-based practice can do to address this in your approach to care. As we have defined evidence-based practice for you in previous chapters, including both what it is and what it is not, we will not cover this explicitly here – only in relation, specifically, to inequalities of health.

The context of health inequalities and evidenced-based practice

Diversity in healthcare is apparent in the patients we care for and the staff delivering that care. However, much of the literature in health education lacks this diversity (Mukwende et al., 2020). To deliver care that is more inclusive and culturally competent we first need to have an awareness of the issues that persist. In an ideal world we would all have the same opportunities and ability to reach our full potential; however, in reality this is sadly not the case. You will have heard the term 'health inequalities' before and are, perhaps, wondering what this has to do with evidence-based practice. Well, health inequalities represent the preventable, inequitable and unjust differences in the status of people's health, alongside the differences in the opportunities and care they receive, which in turn influence their health status (Williams et al., 2022). It is this 'injustice' that Dr Martin Luther King is referring to in his quote above, and it is something we must consider when we look at providing evidence-based practice for our patients and service users. We need to ensure we have considered factors that may affect these individuals to help address some of the issues they may encounter when trying to access care or while receiving care.

Activity 5.1   Critical thinking and reflection

Reflection is used within healthcare as a method of quality improvement and is an essential skill to master. As a nursing associate it's important to look critically at everything we do in order to improve our skills and healthcare provision as a whole and you will also be required to reflect on your activities as part of your NMC revalidation and practice development. It is good to use a reflective model to aid with your reflective practice, as this can help structure the process.

Using your preferred model of reflection, think of the last time you were working in clinical practice and delivered an intervention to a patient.

- Think about the evidence that underpinned this activity.
- Did you carry out the intervention based on what you have been told/shown to do and, if so, did you understand the rationale and evidence behind why you were doing it?
- Do you think there were any needs in relation to age, race, sexual orientation, religion, gender, or disability of the patient that could have been better addressed with more or different research?

If, following your reflection, you recognised that you did not fully understand the evidence-base behind your care, please research this and equip yourself with this knowledge. It is important that we as health professionals can understand the evidence-base behind the care we provide, so that we can help explain care to our patients and we can be assured that the care we are providing is what is in the best interest of the patient. If you felt that there was a gap in the literature then this will provide you with a great learning and discussion opportunity with your peers.

As this answer is based on your own reflections, there is no outline answer at the end of the chapter.

What are health inequalities?

So, what do we mean by the term 'health inequalities'? There are variations in the literature as to what health inequalities are, accounted for to some degree by literature being from outside the UK. You might read some of the literature describing health inequalities as health *inequities*; this is the term the World Health Organization uses to describe the fact that, despite the average life expectancy increasing, this has occurred unequally and with persistent and increasing gaps between those with the best and worst health (WHO, n.d.).

Since we are practising healthcare in the UK, in this chapter we will be referring to health inequalities as *the avoidable and systematic differences in health between groups of people*, as described by the King's Fund researchers (Williams et al., 2022). These differences in health are influenced predominantly by an individual's socioeconomic position and are compounded by other factors such as the nine characteristics protected in law under the Equality Act (2010) (see below), as well as socially excluded groups – for example, people experiencing homelessness and seeking asylum.

Understanding the theory: The Equality Act (2010)

The Equality Act was launched in October 2010 to provide a contemporary and single legal framework to help tackle disadvantage and discrimination. Below is a list of the characteristics protected in law under the Equality Act (EHRC, 2010).

- Age
- Disability
- Gender reassignment
- Marriage and civil partnership
- Pregnancy and maternity
- Race
- Religion or belief
- Sex
- Sexual orientation

Social determinants

It's important to recognise that all our life experiences and circumstances affect our health; these circumstances are called the *social determinants of health*. The social determinants influence health equity in positive and negative ways. Below is a list of those which WHO (n.d.) considers the main influencers:

- income and social protection
- education
- unemployment and job insecurity
- working life conditions
- food insecurity
- housing, basic amenities and the environment
- early childhood development
- social inclusion and non-discrimination
- structural conflict
- access to affordable health services of decent quality.

You will see from this list that these examples are not, strictly, health issues, but are wider factors that have been found to directly impact on a person's health status. Good health, therefore, needs to be considered in terms of 'building blocks' (McGeoch et al., 2023) to help us to recognise a direct link between poor health, health-related behaviours and those who live in the most deprived areas of our country (McGeoch et al., 2023).

This makes addressing health inequalities complex and something that policy-makers have been attempting to address since the early 19th century. The development of the National Health Service (NHS) and welfare state in the first half of the 20th century was predicated on evidence that social inequalities and inadequate access to healthcare were leading to worse outcomes for certain people in society (Acheson, 1998). Despite this, today health inequalities are continuing to widen in the UK, regardless of advances in healthcare and policy aimed at addressing these issues. It is estimated that between 1.3 and 2.5 million years of life are lost due to health inequalities every year (Matheson, 2020).

So let's look at social determinants in more detail. Social determinants of health are defined by WHO as the non-medical factors that influence health outcomes (n.d.). This means that the place you are born and live in, alongside other factors such as economic policies, social policies and political systems all contribute to how you will experience life, with those occupying the lower socioeconomic positions suffering the worst health and outcomes. Life expectancy is itself a key measure of a population's health status. This is due to the systematic relationship between deprivation and life expectancy, which is sometimes referred to as the social gradient (Williams et al., 2022). The social gradient is evidenced by a report by Public Health England (2018a), which found that the difference in life expectancy between the least and the most deprived areas of England was 9.3 years for males and 7.3 years for females, a gap that has not changed in the last decade.

Health inequalities are caused by disparities in the distribution of social, economic and environmental conditions in society and can involve not only differences in life expectancy, but also access to care, the quality of that care, behavioural risks such as smoking and wider determinants of health such as adequate housing (PHE, 2018a; Williams et al., 2022).

Evidence-based practice and health inequalities

Knowledge of what health inequalities are and their impact on individuals is essential for practising health professionals in a bid to reduce the mortality and morbidity of the people for whom you will care as a nursing associate and indeed yourself as an individual. While it is recognised that reducing inequalities is part of a wider sociopolitical issue, health professionals have a very important role in upholding or dismantling systems that continue to widen the health inequalities of individuals. The role of the nursing associate was developed to bridge the gap in clinical practice between clinical support workers and registered nurses in delivering person-centred care in response to the *Shape of Caring Review* (NHS England, 2015), with the *NHS Long Term Plan* (NHS England, 2023a) highlighting the pivotal role healthcare professionals play in promoting health and reducing the impact of health inequalities. This makes it essential that nursing associates are aware not only of evidence-based practice, but also how to deliver this in a way that does not exacerbate health inequalities.

The importance of health professionals having an awareness of wider issues in the context of healthcare cannot be emphasised enough. The ongoing cost of living crisis, for example, means that child poverty alone is predicted to be at its highest by 2027/28 (Francis-Devine, 2023) and, as we've discussed above, social determinants such as these are connected to health inequalities (WHO, n.d.) which represents a significant challenge to healthcare workers.

Perhaps the most obvious and damning example of both health and wider inequalities and their effect on people in recent times is the COVID-19 global pandemic. The pandemic highlighted the pervasive and ongoing effect of inequalities, with ethnic minority groups suffering disproportionate death rates and suffering from worsening non-COVID-related health outcomes (Wade et al., 2022). What is also alarming is that people who are already vulnerable, again due to the determinants of health described above, may receive healthcare that exacerbates these inequalities as opposed to diminishing them (Matthew, 2015). While Matthew writes about healthcare in America, there are certainly comparisons to draw here in the UK. Kapadia et al. (2022), for example, highlight long-standing issues in the experiences and outcomes of ethnic minorities using the NHS, which their report highlights are rooted in structural, institutional and interpersonal racism (Kapadia et al., 2022). Their review, entitled *Ethnic Inequalities in Healthcare: A Rapid Review*, identifies inequalities across a number of different health provisions here in the UK. In relation to maternity services, it identifies poor communication and discrimination as being at the root of some of the inequalities and poor outcomes observed, with Black women 40 per cent more likely to experience miscarriage than white women and four times more likely to die during childbirth. These figures are stark and are not intended to be sensational. Moreover, they are intended to shine a light on the disparities that some members of our society face, so that change may occur. We include a link to the report at the end of this chapter.

As health professionals we need to deliver healthcare in a system that values and utilises the evidence to create healthcare services that address the issues facing our patients. One example of this is a report by NHS England (2018) that highlighted that people with learning disabilities and or autism experience greater difficulties in accessing NHS services and, as a result, have far poorer outcomes than the general population. This comes on the back of reports by Mencap highlighting the number of avoidable deaths of people with a learning disability that have occurred *within* healthcare settings (Mencap, 2007, 2012). More recently, the death of young man with autism, Oliver McGown, highlighted still further the need for all health and social care staff to be appropriately trained to meet the needs of people with a learning disability and autism; this has now been made mandatory as part of the Health and Care Act (DHSC, 2022). Oliver died, not as a result of a medical condition, but because of medication he was given against his own wishes and that of his parents. Oliver died from an adverse reaction to this drug; the subsequent review confirmed that his death had been avoidable (Harris, 2022). As a nursing associate you may already have had what has become known as the 'Oliver McGown Training', as all organisations who are CQC regulated are now required to ensure their staff are suitably trained to meet the needs of this vulnerable group.

Activity 5.2   Critical thinking and reflection

In Chapter 3 we asked you to think about the equipment you use in your place of practice and whether any of it could have been designed better if a service user had been involved. Here, we would like you to consider your workplace as a whole; using the knowledge you have now gained from this chapter so far, consider how accessible you think it is to *all* patient groups.

Use the prompts below to help you.

- Does the layout and information provided exclude any patient group?
- How accessible is the *information* that is available to service users and their families/carers?
- Is there a designated lead for learning disabilities?
- Would you be confident that you could deliver information to meet the needs of hearing- or sight-impaired service users/carers?
- Do you think there are any barriers to service users and carers accessing your services and, if so, how might they be addressed?

An outline answer is provided at the end of this chapter.

Intersectionality

The term 'intersectionality' has its roots in Black feminist activism, and was originally coined by American critical legal race scholar Kimberlé Crenshaw in 1989. Crenshaw used this term to describe the double discrimination of sexism and racism that Black women faced in the legal system. The term is now used to refer to the way in which different and overlapping social identities such as gender, class, race and so on intersect to create multiple layers of discrimination and disadvantage. An example of intersectionality would be a person with a disability, who is also female and lesbian. These separate social identities in and of themselves could lead to health inequalities. However, the existence of them all together puts this person at greater risk, which then, when layered together, can create multiple layers of disadvantage. It goes without saying that this does not only apply to the patients and service users, but also to us as members of staff and users of the health service also. These intersections will influence the way in which you experience working in the health service and indeed navigating the health service yourself. They will also have had a bearing on your life journey to becoming a nursing associate and are likely to impact the way in which you will conduct your practice.

Unconscious bias

As we discussed earlier in the Chapter, the Equality Act (EHRC, 2010) identifies nine characteristics where evidence has shown that significant discrimination still exists towards people who hold any one (or more) of these characteristics and this includes access to and the service they receive relating to their health. Given that these characteristics are protected in law, it would be nice to think that discrimination would not happen. However, as we have learnt so far, this is not the case. Some of the reasons behind this are to do with people not considering the needs of people that have issues they cannot relate to, or they have not thought of, such as the example we gave in Chapter 3 of a building being designed by people without mobility issues without the input from people who do have mobility issues such as wheelchair users. Other acts of discrimination can be the result of unconscious bias. Unconscious bias or implicit bias as it is sometimes referred to, is a way to describe your attitude and association to an individual. This exists outside of your conscious awareness and is something that affects everyone. The way in which you think is dependent on your life experiences, and the beliefs and views you hold around other people. It does not only relate to the protected characteristics identified in the Equality Act (EHRC, 2010), but could include height, weight, names and so on. Unconscious bias can mean that you think about or treat someone preferentially because you are alike, or you have a preconceived idea of this individual; conversely, you could also think about, or treat the person less favourably because of their differences and preconceived ideas of that individual or group of people. These can sometimes be known as *stereotypes*. Everyone can think in a way that involves unconscious bias to a lesser or greater extent, but it is important to be aware of this and to recognise how this could affect your judgement and attitudes towards others. If unconscious bias is to be addressed overall, we need to be aware of our own attitudes and assumptions and take steps to mitigate these.

Activity 5.3   Critical thinking and reflection

Copy the following link into your web browser or search for the Tedx talk called 'How to Outsmart your own Unconscious Bias' by Valerie Alexander.

www.youtube.com/watch?v=GP-cqFLS8Q4

Below is a link to NHS England Leadership Academy. Having watched the video above, use their guide to complete your own unconscious bias training.
https://learninghub.leadershipacademy.nhs.uk/guides/the-impact-of-stereotyping-clark-doll-test/steps/unconscious-bias-suggested-but-needs-refining/
There is no outline answer at the end of the chapter.

The challenges and triumphs

Evidenced-based practice is a way of practising healthcare that standardises practice based on evidence of populations using research, or other systematic approaches, as opposed to using instinct, as clinical practice often did in the past. While this has clearly been an important development for modern medicine and nursing practice, we must continue to apply scrutiny to the research evidence produced and to call for research that engages the appropriate people and asks the appropriate questions to ensure that we are not just learning part of the story. In Chapter 3 we told you of the importance of involving service users and carers as active participants of research. However, in the interest of reducing health inequalities, we should consider to what extent disadvantaged groups participate in the production of research evidence and what can be done to address that, or at least raise this awareness. We must also ensure that we are examining the evidence with criticality, ensuring that it meets the needs of the people we care for.

An example here might be research on the efficacy of digital consultations for people that may be at a disadvantage, such as those who are older in age, of lower socioeconomic status, or those who have limited English proficiency. Digital consultations have seen a significant increase in recent years, in part propelled by the COVID-19 global pandemic. However, the rise in this activity could place some patients at disadvantage; although it is important to continue to develop our care system, and adapt to different models of delivery, we must also be mindful of widening health inequalities for patients, placing them at greater risk (Gray and Sanders, 2020).

Finally, we would like to highlight how some members of our society have been 'left out' of the text books from which we learn – and of the equipment and technology that we use. Caroline Criado Perez coined the phrase 'invisible women' in her best-selling book of the same name (2019; we include it at the end of this chapter in the Annotated further reading section). You may have heard her name in connection with the campaign to have a woman depicted on the back of a British bank note after the Bank of England proposed replacing the picture of Elizabeth Fry with that of Winston Churchill, meaning there would be no historical women of note on a British bank note. In her book she highlights how men are considered the 'default human' within society and how research, and research data, are generally biased in favour of men. Symptoms for stroke, for example, are different in women to men, yet, until recently, it was the symptoms in men that medical students were taught as the default 'normal' symptoms to look out for (Criado Perez, 2019).

An article by Bibbins-Domingo and Helman (2017) highlights how a lack of representation in clinical research risks undermining its overarching goal. An example of where research did not take into account differences can be found in potential racial bias in *pulse oximetry*. Pulse oximeters are a non-invasive way of monitoring a patient's oxygenation, also known as SpO2. Pulse oximeters are required to be tested in a laboratory environment, as with other medical devices, to ensure their validity; however, this testing typically took place on patients with lighter-pigmented skin as a default and therefore they excluded a significant proportion of patients with darker-pigmented skin as standard. It then came to light that – along with other factors for errors and reliability of pulse oximetry readings such as arrhythmia, cold extremities, nail polish, poor fit and so on – skin pigmentation was also a factor in the reliability of some pulse oximeters. Numerous studies have now been carried out to test this hypothesis, and there are variations in the type of probe used and the outcomes of the readings in patients with darker-pigmented skin in comparison to lighter-pigmented skin. Overall, the research highlights that some pulse oximeters may overestimate the oxygenation level at low oxygen states in people with darkly pigmented skin, meaning that a pulse oximeter may state that a person's oxygenation is better than it is at readings between 92 per cent and 96 per cent (Sjoding et al., 2020).

The good news is that, despite it taking some time for this published research to be filtered down to clinical practice, it is now something that is taught to healthcare professionals alongside other factors that may affect pulse oximetry readings. It also means that, as with any of the vital sign observations that are taken by health professionals, they are used alongside other factors to form a whole clinical picture. Possessing this knowledge may help an individual caring for a patient with darkly pigmented skin to have a lower threshold for escalating concerns over low oxygen saturations and has ensured that when these devices are tested that they don't exclude certain groups. A link to the full report by the NHS Race and Health Observatory, *Pulse Oximetry and Racial Bias: Recommendations for National Healthcare Regulatory and Research Bodies* can be found at the end of the chapter under Useful websites.

Activity 5.4   Critical thinking and reflection

Imagine that you are at the start of your shift on a hospital ward and you take over the care of Henry who is a 68-year-old male. Henry is a retired miner who was born in Jamaica and has lived in Britain since the age of 11. Henry has COPD and has been admitted to the respiratory ward with an infective exacerbation of this. At the start of your shift, you do Henry's observations.

Write down the factors that you need to consider when carrying out Henry's observations and the evidence-base behind these.

An outline answer is provided at the end of this chapter.

Chapter summary

We hope that in reading this chapter, and through undertaking the activities, you now have a better understanding of the issues around health inequalities: what they are and how they contribute to the way in which our patients experience and require care. Overall, evidence-based practice is overwhelmingly positive and has helped the advancement of treatments and patient care. However, more research needs to be undertaken to address topics facing minority and marginalised groups in a bid to raise awareness and shape care services to enable them to meet the different needs of different groups of people. Those working in healthcare should be aware of the issues and the evidence behind them. We hope that reading this chapter has made you reflect on your own views and knowledge and has sparked an interest to find out more. Please continue to apply the best available evidence to the care you provide: by applying a level of scrutiny to your own practice you might be able to identify where policies and practices that may exacerbate existing issues exist. You are the future of healthcare.

Activities: Brief outline answers

Activity 5.2 Critical thinking and reflection

It is important to consider the accessibility of your area; we have often been in hospitals and clinical settings where there are multiple items strewn along corridors that could make access more perilous if, for example, you were sight impaired or a wheelchair user.

In considering whether your area excludes any patient group, it is hoped that all the buildings are accessible, but this may not be the case in old or temporary buildings. Accessibility does not only relate to how easy it is to physically navigate the building though. Is signage clear and readable? Would it be understandable to someone whose ability to read English was limited? Or is this provision considered?

Is the environment noisy and chaotic, would it be suitable for someone who is neurodivergent and is this considered in your appointment scheduling? People feeling able to access a service might also be affected by the perceived welcome they receive. This applies to the variety of imagery used in displays as we tend to be biased towards people with whom we can identify ourselves, as discussed previously in the unconscious bias section. If the workforce is not diverse, and someone has not thought about representation, then this can be missed. It also relates to the language used by the staff and that provided in written information. Is the language ableist and heteronormative, for example? If these, or any of the terms you have read, are new to you, please take some time to go away and read up on these and familiarise yourself with them so that you might suggest ways in which your clinical area might make the environment a more inclusive place to both work and receive care.

The accessibility of the information should consider people who do not speak English or those unable to read it and people with a sight impairment. Literature provided should consider the context of different genders and sexual orientations, so that we do not exclude people and prevent them from feeling welcome and seen in our services. In meeting the needs of patients that are hearing or sight impaired we must be able to ensure that information is shared with consent as to how to best meet that individual's needs. Have you heard of the *reasonable adjustment flag*? This was developed in the NHS Spine to enable health and care workers to record, share and view details of reasonable adjustments across the NHS, wherever the person is treated. Here is a link to the website:

https://digital.nhs.uk/services/reasonable-adjustment-flag#:~:text=The%20standard%20 aims%20to%20make,health%20and%20social%20care%20services

Considering the evidence around poor outcomes for patients with a learning disability, the Health and Care Act (DHSC, 2022) set out training that should be completed by all who care for people with a learning disability and/or autism to make sure they meet the standards and deliver the outcomes that people with learning disabilities, autism or both and their families expect and deserve.

I hope that, following your reflection on whether there are any barriers to service users and carers accessing your services, you have been able to reflect on any gaps in your knowledge and indeed in your service so that you can look to work with your colleagues to address this.

Activity 5.4 Critical thinking and reflection

Here is a list of some of the things you might consider.

- *Introductions and infection control*: The evidence for considering how we approach patients was brought to the fore by Dr Kate Granger and her campaign 'Hello my name is'. This, along with other failings in healthcare such as those highlighted in the Mid Staffordshire inquiry, illustrate why it is important that we provide kind and compassionate care to our patients, starting with the introductions.

- *A–E assessment*: When assessing Henry's pallor, as part of your cardio-respiratory assessment, you will be checking for the presence or absence of cyanosis. Cyanosis is the bluish tinge to skin caused by too much deoxygenated blood. There are a variety of causes for cyanosis and these can be broken down into peripheral or central, so the cause would need to be investigated and treated accordingly. Assessing for cyanosis involves checking the skin and mucous membranes for signs of colour change. It is important to be aware that in people with darker-pigmented skin this is less easily detected. An example of where the evidence is changing to help reduce disparities in assessment is that guidance is now given as to how to detect cyanosis in patients with darker-pigmented skin (NHS England, 2023b). When assessing patients with darker skin, cyanosis is more likely to be able to be assessed by checking the soles of the feet or palms of the hand. In a patient with dark-pigmented skin, the presence of central cyanosis may be indicated if the end of the nose goes a white/grey colour instead of blue; also checking the mucous membranes and tongue is better than observing the lips. This highlights that care needs to be individualised, but that awareness of difference needs to be raised to ensure that care is safe and effective for people of all ethnic backgrounds.

- *A–E assessment*: Exposure, when assessing skin integrity, you must be mindful of the signs of tissue damage in darker skin (Wounds UK, 2021). Historically, medical/nursing education has focused on Caucasian skin in the identification and assessment of skin integrity. Through examining how structural racism has impacted people of colour, evidenced-based practice is now more representative of many different patients. As a medical student Malone Mukwende noticed how teaching in medicine focused only on white skin. He went on to co-author the book *Mind the Gap*, a handbook of clinical signs in black and brown skin (Mukwende et al., 2020) to help address the stark gap in medical literature. A link to the website where the book can be viewed is available in the Annotated further reading section below.

- *Observations and pulse oximetry*: Pulse oximeters may overestimate oxygen saturations in people with darker skin in low oxygen states, depending on the type of device used (Bickler et al 2005; Valbuena et al., 2022). Therefore, when assessing a patient's oxygenation status, the whole clinical picture needs to be taken into account and further tests undertaken if required, with an awareness of this issue.

- *Oxygen*: The administration of oxygen should not be withheld for people with COPD (BTS, 2017). Ensure that the appropriate observation scale and oxygen have been prescribed.

Annotated further reading

Criado Perez, C (2019) *Invisible Women*. London: Penguin, Random House.

This book offers a critical insight into the way in which we are often conditioned to see and experience the world with men viewed as the 'default human' and women as either secondary or invisible. From decisions as to which roads should be prioritised for clearing snow to how medical research is funded and carried out, Perez shines a light not only on how women's invisibility can impact on the quality of women's lives, but also how it can impact their longevity.

Mukwende, M, Tamony, P and Turner, M (2020) *Mind the Gap: A Handbook of Clinical Signs in Black and Brown Skin.* London: St George's University. Available at: www.blackandbrownskin.co.uk/mindthegap

This is a handbook of clinical signs and symptoms in black and brown skin that is missing from the discourse in many medical/nursing texts.

Smith, KE, Banbra, C and Hill, SE (2015) *Health Inequalities: Critical Perspectives.* Oxford: Oxford University Press.

This book offers a critical approach to health inequalities, examining links between research and health inequalities in different contexts.

Useful websites

www.health.org.uk/topics/social-determinants-of-health

This website offers a useful resource for evidence and literature relating to social determinants of health.

www.kingsfund.org.uk/publications/what-are-health-inequalities

This website, similarly, offers useful resources for evidence and literature relating to social determinants of health. It also provides a definition, which we have used in this chapter.

www.nhsrho.org/research/ethnic-inequalities-in-healthcare-a-rapid-evidence-review-3/

This link takes you to the review by Kapadia et al. (2022) that we discuss in this chapter. The review looks at a collection of research papers focusing on ethnic inequalities in healthcare.

www.nhsrho.org/research/pulse-oximetry-and-racial-bias-recommendations-for-national-healthcare-regulatory-and-research-bodies/

This link provides more information on the report Pulse Oximetry and Racial Bias: Recommendations for National Healthcare Regulatory and Research Bodies that we discussed in the chapter, as well as access to their full findings.

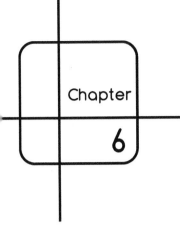

Decision-making in evidence-based practice: The law, ethics and values

Jenny Adams

NMC STANDARDS OF PROFICIENCY FOR NURSING ASSOCIATES

This chapter will address the following platforms and proficiencies:

Platform 1: Being an accountable professional

1.2   understand and apply relevant legal, regulatory and governance requirements, policies, and ethical frameworks, including the mandatory reporting duties, to all areas of practice

Platform 3: Provide and monitor care

3.5   work in partnership with people to encourage shared decision making, in order to support individuals, their family and carers to manage their own care when appropriate

Platform 5: Improving safety and quality of care

5.9   recognise uncertainty, and demonstrate awareness of strategies to develop resilience in themselves. Know how to seek support to help deal with uncertain situations

Chapter aims

After reading this chapter you will be able to:

- recognise and apply underlying concepts and principles of the law, ethics and nursing values relevant to clinical decision-making;
- critically evaluate different approaches when making decisions in complex situations;
- recognise the importance of working with others to improve evidence-based practice.

Introduction

The aim of this chapter is to help you develop strategies to support evidence-based decision-making about care delivery. The NMC *Standards of Proficiency* suggest that nursing associates are expected to 'recognise uncertainty, and demonstrate an awareness of strategies to develop resilience in themselves' and 'Know how to seek support to help deal with uncertain situations' (NMC, 2018b, p. 15). In this chapter we will explore an example of a complex care situation that illustrates the uncertainty and dilemmas faced by nursing associates in applying evidence in practice. Decision-making in practice is not solely based on clinical evidence; you also need to take into account ethics, values and the legal framework governing all medical and healthcare professionals. These requirements are an important part of evidence-based practice. Registered healthcare professionals are accountable in law to their professional body, their employer, the patient and to themselves. This chapter will consider the importance of being able to justify your actions in terms of legal and professional accountability, the patient's preferences and ethical principles. The learning activities we provide, which are based on a case study, will enable you to consider how you work in partnership with other professionals and patients to make safe, ethical, evidence-based decisions.

The case study we present in this chapter is about a nursing home resident, Jim, who lacks capacity to make decisions. Jim's wife, unregistered care staff, the nursing associate, nurses and medical staff are all involved in his care and contribute to decision-making. The decisions discussed in this case study revolve around the current evidence and guidance for pressure area care, Jim's preferences and his lack of capacity to make decisions.

Case study: Jim

Laurel House is a nursing home specialising in caring for older adults with mental health conditions. The nursing home has a culture of person-centred care and prides itself in recognising that all behaviour is a form of communication and expression. The staff are skilled in de-escalation techniques and in communicating with people with dementia.

Jim, aged 78 years, has a diagnosis of dementia. He has lived in Laurel House for three years since his wife was no longer able to care for him at home. There has been an assessment of Jim's capacity to make decisions and give consent. The assessment concluded that Jim had little capacity to make decisions about his own care or to consent to treatment. A liberty protection safeguard authorisation (LPS) is in place to ensure his best interests are met.

Jim is at the end of life and needs palliative care. Jim's wife and the nursing staff believe that Jim thinks of Laurel House as home and has a preference to die in the nursing home.

Jim is bed-bound and prefers to be left quietly to sleep. He has refused to take his medication, including analgesia. He also objects strongly to the care staff carrying out basic care including washing, changing sheets and changing his position. He voices his objections loudly and hits out at staff. Jim seems to be telling staff that everything hurts when he is moved.

The care staff, supported by nurses, respond by disturbing Jim as little as possible. The nurses accept that Jim refuses analgesia, saying he has the right to decide and this decision fits with the policy of person-centred care.

Evidence-based guidelines suggest that you should perform and document regular skin inspections to check areas at risk of pressure ulcers at least once a day, looking out for skin discolouration or soreness. You should also reposition the patient frequently: at last every two hours (DoH, 2015).

One morning the nursing associate does manage to check Jim's pressure areas and observes skin redness on one shoulder and both heels. The nursing associate observes that the skin has broken down over his sacrum.

Later the same day the psychiatrist makes a routine visit. She decides that Jim should be taken to the hospital emergency department by ambulance for IV analgesia and to have his pressure areas treated. This decision is against the wishes of Jim's wife. The nursing staff also believe it is against the wishes Jim would express if he was able to do so.

Activity 6.1   Critical thinking

Nursing associates are still a relatively new profession, closely aligned to that of the registered nurse (RN), with the roles and skills they are permitted to do continuing to expand. With this in mind, read the blog on the NMC website regarding the nursing associate's role (West, 2019).

www.nmc.org.uk/news/news-and-updates/blog-whats-a-nursing-associate/

Next, reflect on your knowledge of evidence-based pressure area care and review the guidance and linked documents to update your understanding. The guidance is available at:

www.gov.uk/government/publications/pressure-ulcers-applying-all-our-health

What do you think the nursing associate's responsibilities are for Jim's care?
There is an outline answer at the end of the chapter.

Legal and professional accountability

The Standards of Proficiency for Nursing Associates, Platform One, 1.2 require you to: 'understand and apply relevant legal, regulatory and governance requirements, policies, and ethical frameworks, including any mandatory reporting duties, to all areas of practice' (NMC, 2018b). The Standard applies to all your activities throughout the working day. As such, you will need to justify your clinical decision-making, demonstrating that your decisions and actions are lawful and work to professional standards, within the protocols and guidance from your employer and meet your patient's needs. You will also need to be personally confident that any decisions you make are not only to the best of your ability, but also to the best evidence that is available. In the following section we will explore this further, considering both professional and legal accountability in decision-making.

Professional accountability

As a registered nursing associate, you will be accountable to your professional body, the Nursing and Midwifery Council (NMC). The purpose of the NMC, which is set out in law, is to protect the public through their functions and activities. These functions include the *registration* of nursing associates, midwives and nurses (i.e. the three professions they regulate); setting standards of education; and undertaking *fitness to practise* processes. Fitness to practise is the name for the system used by the NMC to investigate and apply sanctions for registrants who do not meet the required standards expected. Being a registered nursing associate means you will be required to continue to work to the Code and the Standards of Proficiency (NMC, 2018a, b). If your practice or behaviour falls below the expected standard, the NMC may investigate and apply sanctions (NMC, 2022).

In order to undertake this role, you must be a caring, knowledgeable practitioner who has skills in effective decision-making. The decisions you make as a nursing associate will have an impact on the safety, health and wellbeing of the patient.

The NMC suggests that, as a registered professional, the nursing associate must: 'act professionally at all times and use their knowledge and experience to make evidence based decisions and solve problems' (NMC, 2018b, p. 4). However, in addition to knowledge and experience, effective decision-making also requires skills in critical thinking, analysis and the development of clinical judgement (Holland and Roberts, 2013). These skills will enable you to analyse information from several sources and respond appropriately. As a nursing associate you will work in a complex environment requiring complex decision-making. This is recognised and highlighted by the NMC in the Standards of Proficiency (2018b, p. 3), where it is suggested you will:

> 'work in the context of continual change, challenging environments, different models of care delivery, shifting demographics, innovation and rapidly evolving technologies. Increasing integration of health and social care services will require nursing associates to play a proactive role in multidisciplinary teams'.

The skills in critical thinking and analysis that you develop throughout your training will help your ability to recognise uncertainty and to seek appropriate help and support with complex decision-making.

As well as having the knowledge and skills to provide effective care, as a nursing associate you are also expected to provide safe and competent care and are liable for the actions you take. This means that you are legally responsible for the care you deliver. As such, you need to have an understanding of the law related to nursing associate practice. The law provides another source of evidence on which to base decisions and actions.

Legal accountability

Now that we've provided a bit of context, let's return to the case study regarding Jim. There are several legal issues potentially associated with his care which you may have recognised in your answer to Activity 6.1 above. These issues are:

- duty of care;
- clinical negligence;
- consent;
- mental capacity; and
- best interests.

Let's consider these legal concepts in more detail below.

Duty of care and clinical negligence

The *neighbour principle* underpins the development of current negligence law in the UK. This principle, outlined in the case Donoghue v Stevenson (1932), was laid down in common law. Have a read of it now and note the following quote:

> 'You must take reasonable care to avoid acts or omissions which you can reasonably foresee would be likely to injure your neighbour.'

> Who is my neighbour?

'Persons who are so closely and directly affected by my act that I ought reasonably to have them in my contemplation as being affected ...'

How might this principle apply to your role as a nursing associate? Nursing associates have a duty to take *reasonable care* to avoid acts or omissions in situations when their actions may affect someone. This neighbour principle has been further developed in subsequent legal cases, notably in establishing what reasonable care is using the Bolam Test, following the case of Bolam v Friern Barnet Hospital Management Committee in 1957:

'The standard of the ordinary skilled man exercising and professing to have that special skill'.

The Bolam Test established the idea that a medical professional was not negligent if their actions were consistent with common practice among similar medical professionals and accepted by a reasonable body of medical opinion. Later legal cases refined this definition, but the principle remains unchanged. This principle now equally applies to all healthcare professionals. As such, it is expected that you will undertake care consistent with the standards usually expected of a registered nursing associate. The standard of skill expected, at the point of registration, is laid down in the Standards of Proficiency for Nursing Associates (NMC, 2018b). Equally, you are bound by the Code (NMC, 2018a), which concerns the standards of conduct, performance and ethics for all nursing associates. These two documents outline the standards of care usually expected of you.

In addition, specific clinical activities will also have standards of care underpinned by research and local and national guidance. If most nursing associates of similar levels of experience would apply that specific research or guidance, then that would be considered reasonable care in that specific clinical activity. However, if you don't take reasonable care and someone is harmed by either an action or omission of care, then you would be considered negligent and could be prosecuted under common law.

Consent, mental capacity and best interests

The legal requirement for consent for treatment was confirmed in the case of Airedale National Health Service Trust v Bland in 1993.

'It is unlawful, so as to constitute both a tort and the crime of battery, to administer medical treatment to an adult, who is conscious and of sound mind, without his consent'.

Consent to treatment means a person must give permission before they receive any type of medical treatment, test or examination. In order for a person to give valid consent it must be:

- *voluntary*: the decision to either consent or not to consent to treatment must be made by the person and must not be influenced by pressure from medical staff, friends or family;
- *informed*: the person must be given all of the information about what the treatment involves, including the benefits and risks, whether there are reasonable alternative treatments and what will happen if treatment does not go ahead;
- *capacity*: the person must be capable of giving consent, which means they understand the information given to them and can use it to make an informed decision.

The practitioner should 'take reasonable care to ensure that the patient is aware of any material risks involved in any recommended treatment, and of any reasonable alternative or variant treatments'.

(Montgomery v Lanarkshire Health Board, 2015)

As a nursing associate you should assume that adults are capable of making an informed choice about their care and treatment unless it has been proved that the individual does not have the mental capacity to do so. In order to make an informed choice the adult must have been given the information about benefits and risks involved in the care or treatment in a way that they can understand. The principle requiring practitioners to discuss risks and benefits of any intervention was laid down by the Supreme Court in 2015 in the case of Montgomery v Lanarkshire Health Board. The Supreme Court also gave three situations where the requirement to share information could be waived. These are if the medical practitioner reasonably considers the information would:

- 'be seriously detrimental to the patient's health';
- the patient needs urgent treatment but is either unconscious or has a condition that means that they are not able to give valid consent; or
- the patient may choose that they wish to remain uninformed once have had the opportunity to discuss risks and benefits.

(Montgomery v Lanarkshire Health Board, 2015)

An adult may choose to withhold consent and this decision must be respected even if you don't think it would be wise.

Consent can be given in different ways:

- it may be implied, as in the example of a patient holding out their arm when you ask if you can take their blood pressure reading;
- it may be given verbally – for example, when you ask if you can take a blood sample and the patient says 'yes'; or
- a more formal written consent may be required for more invasive procedures, such as a surgical intervention.

An individual may have a fluctuating capacity to make decisions, which means that their ability to understand or retain information may vary over time or in different situations. If the individual has fluctuating capacity this further complicates the nursing associate's responsibility to seek informed consent. In this situation the person must be supported to be involved in the decision-making process.

In the case study we provided at the start of this chapter, we described someone who lacked capacity to make decisions. If an adult lacks capacity to make decisions about their care, then care and treatment decisions can be made in their best interests, essentially depriving the individual of their liberty.

Deprivation of Liberty Safeguards (DoLS) were introduced in the Mental Capacity Act (2005) to protect adults aged over 18 who have some deprivation of liberty. In England, the local authority is the *supervisory body* that may authorise a deprivation of liberty (DoL) to be put in place in order to carry out treatment or care. The supervisory body must ensure that the required assessments have been done by two separate, suitably qualified professionals (Age UK, 2023). The individual must be consulted, and the assessor must ensure support is in place to help the individual to contribute. Anyone who has been named by the individual must be consulted, along with carers, family and friends or anyone concerned over the individual's welfare, this includes someone appointed under an enduring or lasting power of attorney or a Court of Protection-appointed deputy.

As a nursing associate you would need to ensure all care you provided was in the person's *best interests care plan* and, as far as possible, reflected the person's wishes in line with the Mental Capacity Act (2005). Consulting the patient, carers and others is also in line with the NMC Standard 3.5 to 'work in partnership with people to encourage shared decision making, in order to support individuals, their family and carers to manage their own care when appropriate' (NMC, 2018b). Information about the person's wishes, feelings, values and beliefs in relation to the specific decision should be gathered from carers, friends and family and, if they are involved, advocates, attorneys and their deputies. The aim is to find out and to understand the person's decision-making history (NICE, 2018).

Understanding the theory: Key terms

Below we have provided you with some of the most appropriate, relevant, terms that you will need to understand in relation to DoLS and LPS:

Advanced Care Planning (ACP): ACP is a voluntary process of person-centred discussion between an individual and their care providers about their preferences and priorities for their future care (NHS England, 2022). The discussions may result in: an *advance statement* – of wishes, preferences and priorities – and may include nomination of a named spokesperson, which is not legally binding.; an *advance decision to refuse treatment* (ADRT), which is legally binding; or a *context-specific treatment recommendation* or *decision about care*.

Appropriate person: This is a family member or someone else close to the person, if they are willing and able, who can represent and support the person through the process.

Age assessment: To confirm aged 18 or over.

No refusals assessment: To confirm there is no conflict with another existing authority about decision-making.

Mental capacity assessment: To establish mental capacity to decide on the specific decision.

Mental health assessment: Authorisation can only be given if a mental disorder within the meaning of the Mental Health Act 1983 exists.

Eligibility assessment: If the individual is subject to the Mental Health Act 1983 and detained (*sectioned*), or is subject to a requirement, such as living in a particular place, that would conflict with the DoL.

Best interests assessment: It must be established whether it is in the individual's best interests/ necessary to keep them from harm, and a proportionate response to the likelihood and seriousness of that harm.

Court of Protection: The Court of Protection is based in London. Most cases are heard by district judges and a senior judge, but can sometimes be heard by High Court judges. Cases can sometimes be transferred to a local court for hearing. The Court makes decisions on financial or welfare matters for people who can't make decisions at the time they need to be made (they 'lack mental capacity'). The Court is responsible for making decisions about when someone can be deprived of their liberty under the Mental Capacity Act. It is responsible for deciding whether someone has the mental capacity to make a particular decision for themselves. The Court is also responsible for appointing deputies to make ongoing decisions for people who lack mental capacity; giving people permission to make one-off decisions on behalf of someone else who lacks mental capacity; and handling emergency applications where a decision must be made on behalf of someone else without delay. The Court also makes decisions about a lasting power of attorney or enduring power of attorney and considers any objections to their registration, considering applications to make statutory wills or gifts.

Lasting power of attorney (LPA): Someone with LPA is legally appointed to make decisions on behalf of someone else, if the latter loses mental capacity. It is usually someone close to the person such as a family member or close friend. There are different types of lasting power of attorney. For financial and property decisions, this is known as *lasting power of attorney for financial affairs* in England and Wales, *continuing power of attorney* in Scotland and *enduring power of attorney* in Northern Ireland. For health and welfare decisions, this is known as *lasting power of attorney for health and care decisions* in England and Wales and *welfare power of attorney* in Scotland. It's not currently available in Northern Ireland.

(Continued)

(Continued)

Liberty protection safeguards (LPS): This is a new system designed to provide protection for people aged 16 and above who are or need to be deprived of their liberty in order to enable their care or treatment and lack the mental capacity to consent to their arrangements. It applies to those with conditions like dementia, autism and learning disabilities. LPS were introduced in the Mental Capacity (Amendment) Act 2019: LPS, but had not yet been implemented, by the time this book went to press.

Mental Capacity (Amendment) Act 2019: This is the Act that introduced LPS, which will eventually replace the DoLS system.

Supervisory body: This body organises the assessments needed under DoLS and ensures that there is sufficient evidence to justify a case for DoL; if there is it authorises it.

Activity 6.2   Critical thinking and reflection

Think back to the case study about Jim at the start of the chapter. In relation to the case study, do you believe the nursing staff have met their responsibilities in terms of:

1. clinical negligence?
2. duty of care?
3. consent?
4. mental capacity and best interests?

An outline answer is provided at the end of this chapter.

Working in partnership with others

As well as understanding and applying the legal framework to your work as a nursing associate you should also be aware of the best practice expected of you in regard to ways of working with colleagues and patients. The Code (NMC, 2018a) sets out the standards of conduct and behaviour for all professionals on the NMC register. Several sections within the Code outline an expectation that you will work in partnership with others to deliver safe and effective care. This partnership includes the patient, families, your employer and other members of the multidisciplinary team (MDT). Working with patients and other members of the MDT will ensure that care, based on research evidence, is effective and acceptable to individual patients.

Healthcare workers are also accountable to their employer, who sets out their expectations of staff in policy, guidance and employment contracts. You must ensure you work within this policy to ensure that your employer holds vicarious liability and valid professional indemnity in the event of a claim against the employee (NMC, 2020b).

Person-centred care

The NMC Standard 3.5 says that a nursing associate should 'work in partnership with people to encourage shared decision making, in order to support individuals, their family and carers to manage their own care when appropriate' (NMC, 2018b). This section considers how working with the patient and family can improve outcomes for evidence-based care delivery, but may also create dilemmas when evidence-based interventions are in conflict with the patient's preferences.

The first professional standard described in the Code is 'Prioritise people' (NMC, 2018a); it details the behaviours required to treat people as individuals, to listen and respond to their preferences and concerns. Further guidance on implementing the Code describes person-centred care as thinking about what makes each person unique, and doing everything you can to put their needs first. There is an emphasis on 'working with' rather than 'doing to' (NMC, 2020a). It is believed that understanding the patient's beliefs and values and sharing decision-making can result in better patient involvement, satisfaction with care and a feeling of wellbeing (McCormack and McCance, 2010; NMC, 2020a).

As a nursing associate you must be sufficiently knowledgeable to respond to the individual's physical, social, psychological, spiritual and cultural needs within your own competence and role boundaries (McCormack and McCance, 2010; NMC, 2020a).

In the case study the nursing staff place high value on delivering person-centred care and the nursing home prioritises person-centred care. However, McCormack and McCance (2010) suggest that there are a number of different elements in the care environment that influence the delivery of person-centred care, including organisational systems and the potential for innovation and risk-taking. The local authority has considerable influence over these elements of the nursing home environment and will not permit the nursing home staff to administer IV medication if there are no medical staff based on-site. In this example, therefore, it limits the physical care the nursing staff can offer.

Activity 6.3   Critical thinking and reflection

Watch the NMC's animation 'Let's talk about person-centred care' from their *Caring with Confidence: The Code in Action* series. You can find it on YouTube here:

www.youtube.com/watch?v=rM9QAxFSBMU

Consider the nursing associate role in delivering person-centred care. Is there ever a conflict in delivering person-centred care and ensuring that care is evidence-based?
An outline answer is available at the end of the chapter.

Working with the multidisciplinary team

The Code (NMC, 2018a) makes it very clear that you must work cooperatively with colleagues to provide effective evidence-based care. Other members of the team will have knowledge and expertise that could improve the outcome for a patient.

In most situations the care of a patient is shared with others and, as such, you must ensure that colleagues are kept informed of the patient's condition and of any changes in care. Sharing information helps to identify and reduce risk.

It is particularly important that others are consulted when that patient does not have capacity to make decisions about care and decisions are made in the patient's best interests (NICE, 2018).

In caring for Jim in the case study, the nursing home staff did consult Jim's wife and referred back to the preferences previously expressed by Jim, but it is not clear if they consulted medical staff – for example, the GP or Jim's psychiatrist. The medical staff could have offered alternative expertise and advice. For example, it may have been possible to administer Jim's analgesia covertly, disguising the medicine in food or drinks. However, this decision must be taken in consultation with the MDT. The Care Quality Commission (CQC) is the inspectorate for care homes and provides clear guidance regarding covert administration of medicines, working within the Mental Capacity Act 2005 (CQC, 2022). This includes holding a best interests meeting and ensuring that covert administration is specifically identified for each medicine prescribed. The pharmacist should also be consulted to confirm that the medication will still be safe and effective if administered in this way.

The CQC suggests that it is only necessary to administer medicines covertly if a person actively refuses their medicine; that person is judged not to have the capacity to understand the consequences of their refusal (as determined by the Mental Capacity Act 2005); and the medicine is deemed essential to the person's health and wellbeing.

Jim does appear to fall into this category. Working with the MDT to find a way to administer Jim's prescribed analgesia could be the key to improving his wellbeing.

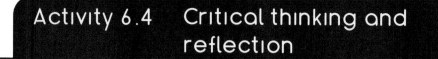

Activity 6.4   Critical thinking and reflection

Find and read:

> CQC (2022) CQC Medicines: Information for adult social care services. Available at: *Administering Medicines Covertly*, oacp.org.uk

What steps could the care home staff take to ensure patient safety when medicines are administered covertly?

An outline answer is available at the end of the chapter.

Ethical decision-making

The NMC expects nursing associates to apply ethical frameworks to all areas of practice (NMC, 2018b). As we touched on in Chapter 3, ethics is the study of what is morally right and wrong, or a set of beliefs about what is morally right and wrong (Cambridge Dictionary, 2023). Individuals learn these moral principles from their family and community as they grow up, therefore there may be some differences in beliefs about the moral rules of behaviour for distinct groups, communities and cultures.

Nurses, along with nursing associates and other professional groups, have their own professional ethics. Professional ethics apply to how nurses and nursing associates behave and practise and the Code (NMC, 2018a) sets out the expectations for your ethical behaviour and practice. The NMC Standards for nursing associates (2018b) stipulate that when making care/ treatment decisions you should look at what research has shown to be most effective while using your own judgement and experience. Your own judgement is informed by both personal and professional ethical principles and therefore underpins decisions you make about applying research evidence in practice.

Activity 6.5   Critical analysis and reflection

Consider a recent situation from your practice that involved an ethical or complex problem you had to solve.

Identify what decisions you made and the evidence behind them. How did you decide if the decision was morally right or wrong?

Discuss your answers with a registered nurse.

Some points you could consider are outlined at the end of the chapter.

Beauchamp and Childress (2001) provide a more detailed ethical framework based on the principles of *autonomy, non-maleficence, beneficence* and *justice*. The principle of doing good (beneficence) and doing no harm (non-maleficence) have been the basis of medical ethics for thousands of years. Autonomy and justice, however, have only been considered important principles more recently as the intrinsic value of individual decision-making and the need to balance resources within a community have been recognised. Let's consider these in more detail.

Autonomy

Autonomy is the ability to self-rule, without the control or interference of others (liberty) and to take actions based on accurate, meaningful information (agency) (Beachamp and Childress, 2001). Autonomy is a complex concept which may be interpreted in many different ways. Individual autonomy may also be restricted under law – for example, prisoners have their autonomy restricted. Autonomy may also be compromised, for example, by ill health or substance misuse.

In healthcare settings the concept of autonomy is closely linked to informed consent and the capacity to consent. Respect for autonomy requires you to both acknowledge the right for an individual to act according to their personal beliefs and also support and build an individual's ability to act autonomously – for example, ensuring a patient understands the information regarding treatment before making a decision is supporting the capacity to make an informed, autonomous choice.

Non-maleficence

Non-maleficence is considered to mean 'do no harm'. Beachamp and Childress (2001) focus on physical harm such as pain, disability and death. However, other harms such as psychological, social or financial harms could also be included.

Non-maleficence in a healthcare situation can be complex – for example, as we discussed in Chapter 1, administering a medication intended to improve a patient's wellbeing but which also has known side effects that could cause harm. You can avoid the risk of causing harm by ensuring the care you provide is evidence-based and that you work within professional standards.

Beneficence

Beneficence can mean both an action done to benefit others and the moral obligation to act for the benefit of others (Beauchamp and Childress, 2001). Most nursing associates recognise the need for beneficence and have an intention to promote wellbeing, acting for the benefit of those requiring care (NMC, 2018b). However, the benefit of any intervention must be balanced against possible risks. The decision to take an action to benefit the health of an individual can also be complicated by the need to balance the impact on others or society in general.

An ethical term that is commonly used in this context is 'utilitarianism', which means something that benefits the greatest number of people. An example of this approach used in healthcare is immunisation. While immunisation protects most people in the community (a beneficial intervention that benefits a large number of people), it is possible that a small number of individuals may be harmed by it.

Justice

The ethical principle of justice is related to fairness and equality. In the context of healthcare, justice relates to the distribution of resources and access to healthcare. When resources are finite, society and the government must decide on the policies that govern access to healthcare. As a nursing associate, for example, you may find that your practice is restricted by policy, rather than individual patient need.

The National Institute for Health and Care Excellence (NICE) is a national organisation with a focus on cost-effectiveness. NICE uses research evidence to identify the most effective treatments and balance the effectiveness and cost. Using guidance published by NICE helps NHS organisations and practitioners to meet the ethical requirement for justice within a finite resource.

NICE clearly demonstrates the evidence-base used in developing the guidance. For example, the process of developing the guidance related to assessment of pressure ulcer risk in nursing homes can be seen at: www.nice.org.uk/guidance/qs89

Ethical dilemmas

In theory, it may seem straightforward to work in accordance with the professional ethics and values of patient autonomy, non-maleficence, beneficence and justice. However, as a nursing associate, you may find yourself in a situation where there is an ethical dilemma – where some of the principles we have discussed in this chapter are in conflict with each other. NMC Standard 5.9 (2018b), 'recognise uncertainty, and demonstrate awareness of strategies to develop resilience in themselves. Know how to seek support to help deal with uncertain situations', highlights the need for nursing associates to be prepared for making decisions in complex situations.

Let's return to our case study about Jim. Jim previously expressed his desire to stay at home at the end of his life. This was an autonomous decision, made when he had capacity to make that decision. Jim is also currently expressing a desire to be left alone. However, his increasing need for care and analgesia suggest that going to hospital could improve his wellbeing (i.e. beneficence). Decisions taken by medical or nursing staff to benefit an individual can compromise autonomy. For example, the psychiatrist's decision to admit Jim to hospital for analgesia and treatment was taken with the intention of benefiting Jim by reducing his pain, but as this decision was taken against his expressed wish it will reduce his autonomy.

Soofi (2022) suggests that the conflict between the principles of autonomy and beneficence regarding the care of a person with dementia can be solved by considering three different approaches.

1. Consider consent as a process, rather than as a one-time event. Consent should be revisited with the patient frequently as capacity fluctuates and care needs change.
2. Any decision expressed previously when the patient had autonomy should be considered alongside the decision that the patient is currently expressing. On some occasions the more recent decisions may improve the patient's immediate welfare.

3. The patient's previously made autonomous decision should be interpreted in the context of the patient's current condition.

Applying these concepts may reduce the conflict between making an ethical decision and acting in the patient's best interests. Jim is consistently refusing to give consent to any intervention and expressing a preference to be left alone. However, considering Jim's previous decision in the context of his current health would support the need for better analgesia and treatment in hospital.

Activity 6.6   Critical thinking and reflection

Can you identify the ethical principle the registered nurse has prioritised in Jim's care?

As a nursing associate you must be able to apply clinical evidence within an ethical framework. You should be able to justify the decisions you make when implementing the care plan and escalating concerns. Which ethical principles would you apply if you were the nursing associate in the case study?

An outline answer provided at the end of this chapter.

Chapter summary

As a nursing associate you have to make complex decisions when delivering and monitoring care in line with NMC Standard 5.9, 'recognise uncertainty, and demonstrate awareness of strategies to develop resilience in themselves. Know how to seek support to help deal with uncertain situations' (2018b).

While care should be based on research evidence, you must also consider the patient's preferences and holistic needs. You will also need to inform and consult with other members of the MDT involved in the care. Equally, you will need to consider the ethical implications of your decisions and ensure you act within the law, professional guidance and your employer's policies.

However, this isn't always straightforward. For example, in the case study, Jim's physical needs seem to be in conflict with his social and psychological needs. This causes a dilemma for the nursing associate intending to deliver evidence-based, person-centred care in line with professional guidance and the employer's policy. Jim seems to be in pain, saying 'everything hurts' when he is moved, yet he is refusing medication. He refuses to be moved to relieve his pressure areas, preventing the staff from applying the best available evidence in his care, resulting in skin breakdown. His expressed social need is to be left alone and remain in the nursing home with familiar people.

In situations when the research evidence is not clear, or the decision is complicated by other factors, you can justify decisions using a framework of accountability; you are accountable to the law, the NMC, the patient, the employer and colleagues. You are also accountable to yourself and, therefore, you also need to consider the ethical implications of any decision that you make. Careful consideration of these factors can help to support your evidence-based decision-making.

Activities: Brief outline of answers

Activity 6.1 Critical thinking

As an accountable professional caring for Jim, it is the nursing associate's responsibility to:

- provide care as set out in the care plan (in this instance we do not know what was in the care plan);
- monitor care, including:
  - o observing the patient for changes in their condition. Jim appeared in pain and his pressure areas were breaking down
  - o the effectiveness of the intervention. The care was not effective as Jim was not comfortable, stating he was in pain;
- escalate concerns to the registered nurse;
- ensure the registered nurse is aware that Jim is in pain and his pressure areas need further attention;
- record observations and interventions;
- improve safety and quality of care;
- offer to support the registered nurse by contacting the medical team regarding analgesia for Jim;
- consider contributions to audit and organisational policy regarding end-of-life care.

Activity 6.2 Critical thinking and reflection

Duty of care and clinical negligence

The nursing team does have a duty of care to Jim. They could be considered to have failed to do what most ordinary, skilled nurses would do to prevent injury to Jim. However, this isn't clear-cut because the omission of pressure area care might be justified by Jim's expressed preference to be left alone at the end of his life.

Consent, mental capacity and best interests

Jim's lack of capacity to make decisions about his care has been established. The nursing team does support Jim in making decisions as far as possible. However, in this situation an MDT best interests meeting may have identified better ways of ensuring Jim remained pain-free. It is possible that Jim would let the staff attend to pressure area care.

Evidence you might draw on to guide your answers

- Duty of care and clinical negligence
- Bolam v Friern Hospital Management Committee (1957)
- Donoghue v Stevenson (1932)
- NMC, 2018a
- NMC, 2018b
- Consent, capacity and best interests
- Montgomery v Lanarkshire Health Board (2015)
- Airedale National Health Service Trust v Bland (1993)
- Mental Capacity Act, 2005
- Mental Capacity (amendment) Act, 2019

Activity 6.3 Critical thinking and reflection

You may identify several situations when the nursing associate perceives a conflict between delivering evidence-based care and person-centred care.

The patient may not have capacity to make a decision at that moment. Their capacity may fluctuate, they may be too ill or distressed.

The patient may refuse care based on a lack of knowledge and information. The nursing associate has a responsibility to ensure the patient has enough information, presented in a way they understand, to make an informed choice.

There may be cultural or religious objections to a medical or nursing intervention. The nursing associate must support the patient to identify an acceptable course of action. It may be possible to take advice from a suitably qualified person who understands the patient's concerns.

The patient may understand the implications of the decision, but choose a different course of action. Again, the nursing associate must support the individual to find the best possible care that fits with their priorities.

Activity 6.4 Critical thinking and reflection

Read the care home policy on covert medicines administration.

Check there has been a best interests meeting or discussion recorded that included the prescriber, pharmacist and the patient's advocate. The reasons for the decision should be recorded.

Ensure the decision has been recorded in respect of every drug that can be administered covertly.

Check the decision to administer medicines covertly has been reviewed and updated as planned.

Medicines that have been altered by crushing or adding to liquids are administered *off licence* and their effect may be altered. The patient must be observed for possible side effects or overdose.

Medicines administration must be recorded as usual, with an additional note if it was covertly administered. The impact of covert medicines administration on the patient must be recorded.

Activity 6.5 Critical analysis and reflection

Do your beliefs put you in conflict with the beliefs of any patient in your care or with other staff – for example, religious beliefs, beliefs about the right to life or assisted suicide?

Did your personal beliefs influence the care decision you have discussed with the RN?

Professional ethics: Can you identify the section of the Code (NMC, 2018a) that could guide your actions?

Explore *Principles of Biomedical Ethics* (Beauchamp and Childress, 2001), discussed in this chapter, and identify which you would apply to your decision.

Using a professional ethical framework can help you to make decisions that are patient-centred and support the patient's best interests.

Activity 6.6 Critical thinking and reflection

The ethical principle the RN has prioritised in Jim's care is autonomy. The RN has considered Jim's previously expressed view – that he wished to die in the care home. The RN was also supporting his current wish not to have any nursing or medical intervention.

You may decide to balance the ethical position taken by the RN and consider the principles of beneficence – to do good. If this is the principle you choose to prioritise then ensuring Jim has analgesia and pressure area care may improve his wellbeing.

Annotated further reading

McCormack, B and McCance, T (2010) *Person-Centred Nursing: Theory and Practice.* Oxford: John Wiley & Sons.

This book explores the concepts of personhood and person-centredness. It introduces a framework for person-centred nursing based on the nurse, the care environment, person-centred care processes and evaluating the outcomes of person-centred care.

Avery, G (2017) *Law and Ethics in Nursing and Healthcare: An Introduction.* London: Sage.

This is a concise introduction to law and ethics for students and practitioners, helping you to decide 'what is legal' and 'what is right' in order to practise safely and ethically. The book covers key areas such as negligence, consent, confidentiality, and professional conduct.

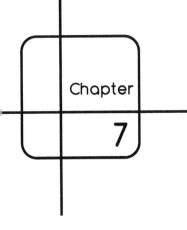

Chapter 7

Change for quality improvement: Putting evidence into practice

Peter Rogers

Chapter aims

After reading this chapter, you will be able to:

- define and explain the concept of quality in healthcare;
- explain some of the drivers of service improvement in healthcare;
- describe some of the commonly encountered change models;
- draw upon your knowledge and understanding to identify, promote and contribute to service improvement projects in your place of work;
- identify your own development needs in relation to service improvement activities.

Introduction

In previous chapters, you will have increased your knowledge and understanding of evidence-based healthcare. You will also have learnt some practical skills, such as database searching and critiquing research, in order to help you better achieve it. In this chapter we take you on the final leg of the journey: how you can be an agent of change in order to improve the quality of the service and care you provide while ensuring that change is evidence-based. As with other chapters in this book, we can't introduce you to everything to do with service improvement, but we include some useful websites and annotated further reading at the end of the chapter to help you build on your knowledge and skills further.

To start, consider the following quote:

Change is the only constant in life.

Heraclitus (c. 535–475BC), ancient Greek philosopher

This is certainly true of healthcare, where our knowledge and understanding of the evidence-base that underpins our practice is constantly developing, as well as the priorities changing. You may recall, for example, that in Chapter 1 we introduced you to Margaret, a retired nurse who trained in the 1950s and was required to wear long sleeves with cuffs and a belt with a metal buckle – neither of which would be allowed in today's healthcare. We talked about *why* practices changed; now, in this final chapter, we are going to talk about *how* change is introduced.

Whether it is new insights gained through research, new treatments made possible by clever inventions, or the novel application of existing knowledge to new problems, the knowledge on which we base our care for and management of those in need is constantly changing. The need for care to be evidence-based is well established (Emanuel et al., 2011; Shuval et al., 2010), and discussed in detail in relation to different perspectives throughout this book. It follows that, in order to continue to provide high-quality evidence-based care, what we do and the way in which we do it *must* evolve along with our understanding of the evidence that underpins our practice. However, changing behaviour is not easy, nor is success guaranteed when we try.

While improvement invariably involves change, change does not necessarily result in improvement.

As we highlight above, the nature of evidence-based practice is addressed more fully elsewhere in this book. The focus of this chapter, therefore, is on the *processes* through which changes in behaviour take place, in order to ensure the practice you provide reflects the current evidence-base.

We will explore the meaning of quality and quality improvement in a healthcare context and how it can be achieved through using a structured approach; we will introduce you to three of the commonest models that are used to organise service improvement projects. As a nursing associate you will not only lead on, but also be involved in change and this chapter will give you the knowledge and understanding to make sense of service improvement initiatives, giving you the confidence to identify opportunities to improve the quality of care provision and to actively contribute to projects alongside your colleagues in the multidisciplinary team (MDT).

We will also explore the relationship between change and improvement, along with the importance of benchmarking and measurement in the assessment of the impact of change initiatives. Finally, we will highlight the challenges of sustaining service improvements which you will inevitably be faced with. However, by encouraging a systematic, inclusive and benefits-focused approach to improvement projects, it is possible to mitigate the uncertainty and anxiety often provoked by change, enabling the professional development of the staff involved and achieving the improvements in patient outcomes and experience everyone wants to see.

We will use some real-life healthcare examples to illustrate how the methods outlined have been applied by others in relation to the organisation or delivery of clinical services.

Quality and quality improvement in healthcare

Before starting to think about the process which might lead to improvement in healthcare services, it is important to first consider the nature of what it is we are trying to improve. What does 'quality' mean in relation to healthcare services?

As a nursing associate, like the majority of people who work in the healthcare profession, you will take pride in providing a high-quality service. However, many of us have found ourselves in situations where we have felt the care provided to patients does not always match our standards, despite others feeling it to be perfectly acceptable. This suggests that the concept of quality is somewhat subjective.

Activity 7.1   Reflection

Spend a few moments noting down what you think are the key attributes of high-quality care.
As this activity is based on your own reflection, there is no outline answer provided at the end of the chapter.

The nature of quality in healthcare

While learning to be a nursing associate, the quality of what you do will be measured against programme and module learning outcomes, the Standards of Proficiency for Nursing Associates (NMC, 2018b) and the Code (NMC, 2018a). However, according to the Health Foundation (Jones et al., 2021), there is no commonly accepted definition of quality in relation to healthcare generally. Nevertheless, healthcare systems around the world are committed to striving to continuously improve the quality of the care they provide and, while a universally recognised definition has yet to emerge, the common *elements* of quality are recognised and provide a focus for service improvement activity wherever it is taking place.

In England there is now a single shared view of quality, as shown in Figure 7.1, which was developed by the National Quality Board (NQB) (2021) and has been proposed as the single definition around which quality improvement activity in England can be organised. Formed in 2009, the NQB champions the importance of quality and drives system alignment of quality across health and care on behalf of NHS England. The core of the model was set out in 2008 by the then health minister and surgeon Professor Lord Darzi in the final report on the government-commissioned review of the NHS (DoH, 2008). It identified three key elements of quality:

- *patient safety*: freedom from avoidable harm;
- *effectiveness*: care and treatment is evidence-based and produces the desired benefits to recipients; and
- *patient experience*: encompassing personalisation, compassion, dignity and respect.

Sometime later the NQB combined these elements, regarded as the things that matter most to those using healthcare services, with two factors related to the *context* within which care is delivered. This became the *single shared view of quality* first published in 2016 and reviewed in 2021 to emphasise the expectation that personalised high-quality care should also be *equitable* and thus fairly available to all who need it and of comparable quality, regardless of any characteristics of the recipient of care.

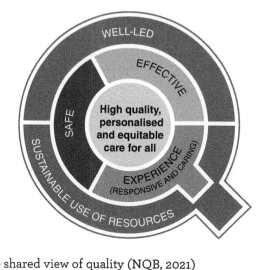

Figure 7.1   A single shared view of quality (NQB, 2021)

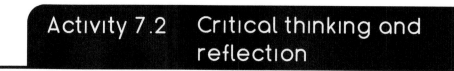

Activity 7.2   Critical thinking and reflection

Reflect on your experience of clinical practice and identify two to three aspects of care which exemplify each of the core elements of high-quality personalised care below:

- safe
- effective
- patient/client experience.

An outline answer is provided at the end of this chapter.

Contextual factors

It is likely that your own focus, and that of colleagues, might primarily be the safety, effectiveness and nature of the patient's experience of the care they receive. However, there will be *contextual* factors (for example, availability and use of resources, and the quality of leadership) that can have a significant impact, positive or negative, on the quality of patient care you provide, and the success or otherwise of any efforts you make to improve care quality. We will return to contextual factors later; however, before moving on have a go at Activity 7.3.

Activity 7.3   Critical thinking

The 'sustainable use of resources' is a broad term that is used and includes workforce planning, staffing, efficiency and finance management in the context of service improvement. While some of these can seem very removed from what you do, you will probably be familiar with the term 'efficiency'.

Again, reflect on your experience of practice and identify two to three examples of where waste or inefficiency could be avoided.

An outline answer is provided at the end of this chapter.

What do we mean by quality improvement?

A reasonable response to this question would be 'anything that makes any or all of the components of the single shared view of quality better'. However, although this answer captures the intended outcome of quality improvement initiatives, it does not help us to understand the underlying processes through which improvement is delivered. Understanding the process is important because it has an impact on the success of any project aimed at improving services. The failure rate of change projects is a topic of debate, but in industry it is generally reported to be as high as 70 per cent (Beer and Nohria, 2000). Fortunately, the situation in healthcare is much better. However, according to the NHS Institute for Innovation and Improvement (NHSI, 2007a) around one in three projects still fail to deliver their anticipated benefits. For NHS information technology projects, the failure rate is around 40 per cent (Cave et al., 2010).

One way to reduce the risk of failure is to use a *systematic approach* to the implementation of change (Wensing et al., 2020, p. 45). Others also emphasise the need to adopt a *systematic* and *coordinated* approach, which uses specific methods to implement changes that deliver demonstrable improvement (Jones et al., 2021 p. 3). Øvretveit (2009, p. 8) goes as far as to incorporate a systematic approach into his definition of healthcare quality improvement; he describes it as 'better patient experience and outcomes achieved through changing provider behaviour and organisation through using a systematic change method and strategies'. While reflecting the importance of using systematic methods to achieve improvement, others also emphasise the continuous nature of service improvement *activity* (Greater Manchester Health and Social Care Partnership, 2018).

Let's break this down further.

The improvement equation

While knowing *how to* make change happen is clearly essential, it is only one of several elements that must come together to produce a demonstrable improvement in service quality. The improvement equation shown in Figure 7.2 offers a high-level overview of the change process and we will use this to organise what follows in this chapter.

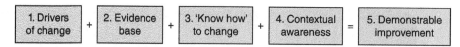

Figure 7.2 The improvement equation

Drivers of change

You may already have heard of the term 'drivers of change'. *Drivers* are the stimulus – the reasons we have for doing something, whatever that something is. In our personal lives it might be a desire to feel comfortable in our favourite pair of jeans which provides the stimulus for us to lose weight. As a nursing associate, the consequences of not meeting your revalidation requirements is likely to provide the motivation to keep you up to date with your continuing professional development. As these examples highlight, drivers can take the form of a benefit, such as being comfortable in our clothes, or the avoidance of a dis-benefit – not meeting the eligibility criteria for re-registration and perhaps losing your job.

Whatever form a driver takes, it provides the *impetus*, the motivation, to change what we do, the way we organise it, or possibly both (Øvretveit et al., 2012).

Activity 7.4   Critical thinking and reflection

- Start by writing down some of the issues where you work that you would like to see change (improvement).
- Next, identify the drivers for change against each of these issues.

Then note down where these drivers originate. Do they come from inside or outside your own team? If it is outside, then consider whether it comes from inside or outside your organisation.

- Finally, identify if these drivers address quality issues (safety, effectiveness or patient experience), or are they more to do with efficiency and cost control?

As this activity is based on your own reflection, there is no outline answer provided at the end of the chapter.

From completing this activity, you will, hopefully, have recognised that some drivers for change are within your control and others are outside it. Those that are outside can be described as *high-level drivers*. These often reflect changes in government policy which are then disseminated and monitored by NHS England and its various departments. The introduction in 2022 of integrated care systems (ICS) following publication of the NHS *Long Term Plan* (NHS England, 2019) and the national COVID vaccination programme are recent examples of such change.

Of course, we are not interested here in the reconfiguration of the NHS in England, or other national initiatives, but rather the local service improvements that take place within health service providers – the things that you, as a nursing associate, will or could be involved in (or indeed lead on). This might include change that is driven by local commissioning priorities, the organisation's strategic plans or by a care provider's internal quality assurance mechanisms. Change at this level might include the merger of services to improve efficiency and effectiveness; action to improve service users' experience based upon reported concerns and complaints; or the remedial action necessary to ensure patient safety in response to the results of routine clinical audit or the root cause analysis of serious clinical incidents.

Evidence-based

Once the drivers for change are identified, the next step in the improvement process is to agree how things can be made better. As you'll know from reading this book, healthcare in general – and medicine and nursing (including nursing associates), in particular – place great emphasis on practice being evidence-based. We have discussed what this involves in earlier chapters in this book, but in the context of this chapter what is meant by evidence-based practice can be described by what is known as the Sicily Statement.

Understanding the theory: The Sicily Statement

This is an agreement, or consensus, which emerged following an international conference of evidence-based healthcare educators and developers held in Sicily in 2003.

Evidence-Based Practice requires that decisions about health care are based on the best available, current, valid and relevant evidence. These decisions should be made by those receiving care, informed by the tacit and explicit knowledge of those providing care, within the context of available resources.

(Dawes et al., 2005, p. 4)

Hopefully, you can see how the Sicily Statement echoes the nursing and nursing associates professions' emphasis on a person-centred approach to care, in which clinical evidence combined with individual expertise and an understanding of the patient's or client's preferences informs the care provided to the individual.

The Sicily Statement goes on to emphasise the need for all healthcare professionals to understand the *principles* that underpin evidence-based practice, not least so that they are able to critically reflect on the basis for the care they themselves provide and therefore ensure what they are doing reflects best practice.

Knowing how to change

As we highlighted above, using a systematic approach is important when implementing a service improvement project, as it will ensure it is more likely to succeed. You may already be familiar with this concept in relation to the nursing process, which has used an established systematic approach to organise person-centred care since the mid-1970s.

Systematic approaches to organising service improvement projects come in the form of change *models*. Models, whether physical or abstract, are simplified representations of something which can help us to understand the more complex thing they represent. There are a number of change models in use within the healthcare sector, which as well as helping people to understand how things can be changed also provide a framework that helps in the planning and delivery of change projects, as well as the communications between the various interested parties to the change.

At a personal level, understanding of the change process will help you, when directly involved in change, to make sense of what you are experiencing and may even give you the confidence to play an active part in the process.

Here we are going to consider three change models which are popular in healthcare improvement projects (Mahmood, 2018; NHSI, 2007a, b and c):

- Kurt Lewin's Change as Three Steps (CATS), commonly referred to as Unfreeze – Change – Refreeze;
- John Kotter's eight-step change model;
- The Model for Improvement, also known as the Plan-Do-Study-Act (PDSA) model.

Lewin's change model

Kurt Lewin was one of the first people to set out a systematic explanation of how planned change comes about. His model is made up of three steps: Unfreeze – Change – Refreeze (Figure 7.3), and is believed to have been inspired by how a block of ice can be melted and the water refrozen into a different shape. It also provides the foundation for many of the change models which followed and which you may also come across (Cummings et al., 2015). Let's have a look at it in more detail.

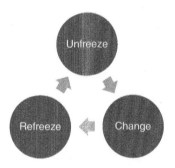

Figure 7.3 Lewin's change model: Change as Three Steps (CATS)

Source: Adapted from Lewin's three-stage process (1951) and Burnes (2004).

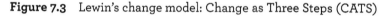

Step 1: Unfreeze

The first step involves ensuring that people recognise the need for change and are prepared for it. Many people are naturally reluctant to change and will understandably push back when what they do, or the way that they do it, is questioned. If people do not understand what is driving the change, they can feel threatened and become resistant to the proposed changes. The first step to mitigate against this reaction is for those promoting the change to make a *compelling case* which sets out the vision for the new future state and the anticipated benefits it will bring. A communication plan helps to ensure that all of those who will be directly affected by the planned changes, as well as those with a peripheral interest in the service, are fully aware of the case for change and are kept informed of the progress of the project.

You may be able to relate, from your own experiences, to the fact that the prospect of change can cause anxiety for those affected by it. However, linking the proposed changes to shared professional or organisational values, like a commitment to providing high-quality care or effective team working, can help to overcome the resistance that can come about from uncertainty. Having a clear project plan that sets out what should happen and when also helps to remove any confusion.

Activity 7.5   Critical thinking

There are many examples of change that have taken place in the UK across the years. Some examples of these include road safety initiatives, such as the compulsory wearing of seatbelts in cars, and cultural changes, such as the wearing of helmets by cyclists. Equally, there will be many that have been introduced within the health service itself.

Let's return to look again at our nurse, Margaret, from the 1950s. What might have been included in the compelling case to abolish the wearing of buckles on nurses' uniforms, such as the one that Margaret had to wear?

An outline answer is provided at the end of this chapter.

Step 2: Change

Once the case for change has been made the process of making the transition from the current state to the desired new future state can commence with the implementation of the *project plan*. The project plan is the document often presented as a Gantt chart (a visual step-by-step list of what needs to be done, laid out as a timeline) that sets out in chronological (date) order the actions required to deliver the desired change. It identifies the anticipated start and end dates for the various activities; any dependencies between actions – for example, 'A' must be achieved before 'B' can commence; and the milestones or key steps that need to be completed as the project moves forward.

In considering what actions need to be taken to bring about a change, Lewin advocated the use of something called *force field analysis* (Thomas, 1985). Lewin proposed that the current state of any situation (the status quo) is the result of a dynamic equilibrium which exists between the forces pressing for change and the forces resisting it. If change is to occur this balance has to be *disrupted* either by increasing the forces driving change or diminishing the forces resisting it, or by doing both. A force field analysis can help those trying to implement change to determine not only what action to take to boost the drivers or diminish the forces resisting change, but also to understand the relative importance of those actions in achieving the desired new future state.

Consider the following scenario. Although this wouldn't be a service improvement project that you might lead on as a nursing associate, it might well be one that you find yourself *experiencing*.

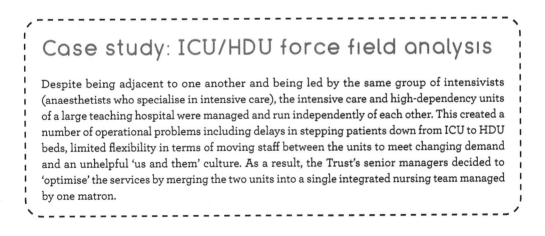

Case study: ICU/HDU force field analysis

Despite being adjacent to one another and being led by the same group of intensivists (anaesthetists who specialise in intensive care), the intensive care and high-dependency units of a large teaching hospital were managed and run independently of each other. This created a number of operational problems including delays in stepping patients down from ICU to HDU beds, limited flexibility in terms of moving staff between the units to meet changing demand and an unhelpful 'us and them' culture. As a result, the Trust's senior managers decided to 'optimise' the services by merging the two units into a single integrated nursing team managed by one matron.

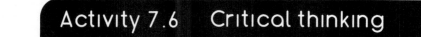

Activity 7.6   Critical thinking

Read the case study and consider the diagram (Figure 7.4) below.

Spend some time thinking about what you think the main drivers for change were and what you think might be the factors resisting the change.

Think about the relative importance of the factors and write what you think are the most significant factors on either side against the largest arrow (or just give one + for the least important and up to three +s for the most important in your notes).

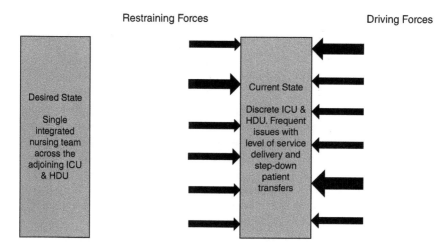

Figure 7.4   Force field example: ICU/HDU optimisation

Factors that you may have considered are discussed later in this chapter.

Step 3: Refreeze

The final stage in the model is associated with a return to stability as a new equilibrium is established. The successful transition is celebrated and the new ways of working are integrated into 'business as usual'; where appropriate this is captured in policies, procedures and care pathways. The change becomes part of 'the way we do things here'.

Rather than see the last step in Lewin's model as a time of necessary consolidation, some critics think 'refreezing' suggests a degree of permanency that is out of step with the pressure for continuous improvement in modern organisations (for example, Child, 2015, p. 350). However, if changes are not allowed to bed in and their benefits given time to materialise those involved become disillusioned and confused and less inclined to engage with subsequent improvement initiatives. As well as being counterproductive, it is also unnecessary. Remember Lewin's inspiration: anything that is frozen can always be unfrozen and reshaped again and again as circumstances demand.

John Kotter's eight steps for leading organisational change

Now let's look at a second model for service improvement, which has more steps involved in it.

Kotter's model (Kotter, 2012) was developed to help organisations overcome what he had observed to be the eight main barriers to the successful implementation of change in organisations, so let's go through each of these now in turn.

Step 1: Create a sense of urgency

This first step focuses on developing and presenting a case for change which enables others to appreciate the need for immediate action. The drivers, as we've discussed above, are used to make a compelling case for immediate action. This first step is sometimes described as creating a *burning platform*. In other words, making others *want* to jump off it.

Step 2: Build a guiding coalition

Leading change is easier when the responsibility is shared within a team. Therefore, in this next step, Kotter advocates building a coalition of people committed to the change who have the complementary knowledge, skills and experience necessary to drive the project forward, persuading the reluctant, coordinating activity and delivering the accompanying communication strategy.

Step 3: Form a strategic vision

This involves using the varied talents of the guiding coalition, as created in Step 2, to set out an understandable and inspirational vision of what the future state will look like, how it will be different from the current state and the 'road map' to its achievement.

Step 4: Communicating the change vision

Kotter makes the point that organisational change, particularly large-scale change, needs a critical mass of people to rally to the cause and sign up for what the change entails. In order for that to happen the vision needs to be communicated widely, clearly and frequently using every available channel within the organisation, which is the aim of this step.

As well as describing the vision, it is also important that the guiding coalition of change leaders are accessible to those with questions and concerns. People will have different motives for engaging with a project, and that is fine, but what does matter is that they are committed to moving in the same direction in order to realise the vision. To achieve this, change leaders need to respond to queries in a supportive, honest and transparent way.

Step 5: Enable action by removing barriers

The aim of this step is to identify and take action to remove any barriers that might threaten the success of the project. This could be any number of factors including, for example: staff who cannot respond as required perhaps because of a lack of training; processes such as professional hierarchies which impede interdisciplinary collaboration; or physical limitations such as a lack of equipment.

Step 6: Generate short-term wins

The aim of this step is to achieve some *quick wins*. It often takes time for the benefits of change projects to become apparent, so planning for some quick wins can provide a valuable boost to motivation and reassure those involved, including the sponsors, that the project is on track and the upheaval involved is worth it. Quick wins can also inspire those who were reluctant to sign up to join their colleagues and get involved.

Step 7: Sustain acceleration

While quick wins are important in building momentum, Kotter cautions against complacency and emphasises the need to maintain the sense of urgency created in Step 1. In this step, therefore, the project team use the increased credibility that comes with initial success to push ahead with the plan, initiating change after change until the vision is realised.

Step 8: Institute change

Rather than *introducing* change, which is what all of the earlier steps in the model have been about, what Kotter is referring to in this step is *embedding* change in the organisation's culture. It involves reinforcing the changes and how they link to the vision and reiterating the benefits to the organisation to ensure the new way of working is strong enough to suppress any inclination to revert to past behaviours. This step is about celebrating the success of the process and the contribution of those involved, so fostering a *can do* mentality towards change which will serve as a foundation for future projects.

Lewin's model has been criticised for being too simplistic (Cummings et al., 2015), an observation which at first seems fair when it is compared to Kotter's eight-steps model. However, if you look closely at the two models, the difference between the two is that Kotter's model simply breaks the process down into more detail, rather than proposing a different process. Kotter's Steps 1–3 describe what Lewin called *unfreezing*, Steps 4–7 are concerned with delivering *change* and Step 8 is synonymous with *refreezing*. Kotter's explanation of change can be seen as adding 'flesh to the bones' provided by Lewin and may explain why some change consultants advocate using the two models together (Tanner, 2022; Watson, 2017).

Model for Improvement

The final model we are going to introduce you to is the Model for Improvement, which has its roots in the work of W. Edwards Deming, an American engineer and academic who became recognised as an expert in the field of quality improvement. At the centre of the model is the *PDSA cycle* developed by Deming in 1993 (Moen and Norman, 2009). The PDSA cycle provides a systematic approach to continuous quality improvement based on what is called the *scientific method of enquiry* and is used a lot in industry.

In 1996 Langley et al. merged the PDSA cycle with three questions to create the Model for Improvement (Figure 7.5). The model was promoted by the Institute for Healthcare Improvement (IHI) in the US for use in health-related service improvement projects and was subsequently adopted by the NHSI (2007b) within the United Kingdom. Figure 7.5 provides a visual model of its different parts.

The first part of the model is made up of three questions to provide clarity about the purpose and approach to the improvement project before the testing of new ideas starts. The answers to question 1 should clearly specify the aims and objectives of the project, with the answer to question 3 setting out the actions required to fulfil them. The answer to question 2 should set out how the success of the project will be judged and requires change leaders to identify the measures that will be used to demonstrate whether the project succeeds in delivering the anticipated improvements. It is important to do this before the implementation and testing of any changes because being able to demonstrate positive change invariably requires comparison of the post-implementation position with pre-implementation baseline data.

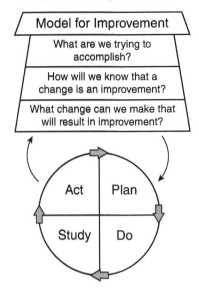

Figure 7.5 The Model for Improvement

Source: Langley et al., 2009. With permission of John Wiley & Sons/Jossey-Bass.

The second part of the model is the PDSA cycle itself, a process which is often repeated multiple times in the testing, refinement and scaling up of potential service improvement actions. The box below provides a more detailed description of each stage.

Understanding the theory: Phases of the PDSA cycle

1. *Plan.* The cycle starts with a plan which includes a statement of the objectives and the rationale for them, followed by the actions designed to deliver them. The statement of the actions, the *what*, is accompanied by an indication of who is responsible for them, as well as *when* and *where* they are expected to be completed.

2. *Do.* The second phase in the cycle is where the plan is carried out. The progress of implementation and any problems or unanticipated observations are documented. Data associated with the changes is collected and the analysis of it starts.

3. *Study.* The study phase of the cycle involves the completion of the data analysis and comparison of the results with the project objectives. The results, along with documented progress notes, are combined into a summary of the learning gained. This new knowledge helps those implementing change to predict where or not the changes they are implementing are likely to work in different circumstances and settings: predictions which can be tested in subsequent PDSA cycles

4. *Act.* This last stage involves deciding, in light of the learning that has taken place, if any changes are required to the plan. If another cycle starts to test the scaling up of the changes, or to test new interventions – or indeed if the changes have failed to deliver the improvement aims – then the plan would need to be dropped and new approaches explored.

(Langley et al., 2009)

While the three models considered here are often presented as separate frameworks, they are in fact complementary. Just as Kotter's model provides more detail to Lewin's description of the change process, the Model for Improvement can be seen as a method for delivering the change step in Lewin's model and hence Steps 4–7 of Kotter's model.

Contextual awareness

The insight gained during the study phase of the Model for Improvement brings two benefits. It enables the change team to decide on the viability of the interventions being implemented, adjusting where necessary to ensure they are effective in achieving the desired aims or, if required, stopping the process and rethinking the planned approach.

The second benefit is that the learning associated with the study phase provides a basis on which change leaders can predict the likely outcomes of implementing changes in different contexts (Langley et al., 2009).

Predictions based upon experience can be useful in gaining support for a new change project; however, evidence-based changes that work in one setting do not necessarily transfer to another (Coles et al., 2020). When changes that worked well in one ward or department fail to gain traction and deliver the anticipated benefits in a different setting the reasons cited are often related to the setting itself – that is, they are *contextual* (Grol and Wensing, 2004).

Activity 7.7   Critical thinking

Although contextual factors are often identified as the problem when something has not gone to plan, they may also facilitate change, which in part explains why introducing the same changes in different settings can have different outcomes.

- What do you think is meant by the term 'contextual factors'?
- Write down five or six examples of what you think could be considered to be important contextual factors in somewhere you currently work or have worked in the past.

An outline answer is provided at the end of this chapter.

The importance of context is acknowledged in the NQB's 2021 version of the single shared view of quality (Figure 7.1). However, as important as they are, there is more to context than just the quality of leadership and the sustainable use (and, one might add, availability) of resources. Øvretveit (2011, p. i18) defines context as 'all the factors that are not part of a quality improvement intervention itself'. While this might seem obvious, it is important not to think of context simply as a backdrop against which change happens. Context is dynamic; its elements can interact with the change process to promote or frustrate the achievement of the improvement aims.

Although the influence of contextual factors in healthcare quality improvement projects has been recognised, our understanding of which factors matter most in different change situations is still developing (Taylor et al., 2011). For example, in the ICU/HDU optimisation example we gave you above part of the context was the availability of overtime and bank shifts to the ICU nurses. The changes being implemented threatened this, which led to some ICU nurses being resistant to the proposed changes. However, no such resistance was encountered from the nurses on the HDU, who had fewer opportunities to earn overtime or take bank shifts as any shortfall in numbers on the HDU was more easily covered by moving staff from other areas.

The fluid nature of the interactions between improvement interventions and the context within which they are being introduced means change leaders must consider how the interactions might play out in each unique setting and plan accordingly (Coles et al., 2020). One way in which change teams can become aware of and so plan their response to the contextual influences on change interventions is to use Lewin's force field analysis to reveal them.

Demonstrable improvement

If the change project has gone to plan, the final result should be the achievement of *demonstrable improvements*.

Demonstrating that the changes implemented have resulted in real improvement requires the measurement of the different elements linked to the aims and objectives of the change project. In other words, there needs to be a *meaningful (measurable) comparison* of the 'before and after'. To do this, a baseline (a measurement of the before) needs to be taken of every different element. To compare this to what you might do in practice, it is like recording a patient's vital signs before they have an operation, so that when you record them post-operatively you have something to compare them to. This is why most improvement projects start with the collection of data rather than implementing change.

Deciding what to measure requires consideration of a number of factors. Have a look at the information in the following box to help you understand better what these might be.

Understanding the theory: Measurement considerations

The type of data to be collected.

- Exactly what data is required to judge whether or not the project objectives have been achieved? Carefully defining what measures are needed helps to avoid the collection of irrelevant data, which is a waste of resources.
- Will the data be quantitative or qualitative? The type of data collected can have a big impact on the work required to report it later. The challenge with numerical data may be limited to how best to present it, whereas qualitative data – for example, narrative responses to a questionnaire or recordings of interviews – may require analysis to identify themes within the data. As you'll have seen from Chapters 3 and 4, as well as being time-consuming this requires particular skills, and possibly the use of dedicated software.

How will it be collected?

- Is the data already being collected within the organisation, or will it require a new process to be agreed and established? Being able to use data already collected as part of the organisation quality assurances processes, such as clinical audit, can save a great deal of effort. It can also speed up the project as the baselines may, in effect, have already been established.

How much pre-change data is required?

- How much data is needed to establish a useful representative baseline? Does the service experience cyclical differences which need to be incorporated into the baseline data – for example, the demand for urgent care services at seaside resorts in the summer?

(Continued)

(Continued)

Setting targets

- Some improvement aims may contain or imply a specific target to be achieved – for example, 'all elective admission for orthopaedic surgery will have a pre-admission assessment'. In this case change leaders, aware of the baseline data, will need to decide if this should be the target from the outset of the project or if an incremental approach in which intermediate targets are set is more likely to be successful ultimately.
- Targets that are too ambitious are demoralising and leave the change team feeling frustrated. A staged approach can build confidence and the belief that success is achievable.

Presenting the data

- Make the data easy to understand by keeping the presentation as simple as possible. Have a look at the example in Figure 7.6 below. The chart contains the same data; which do you find the easiest to interpret?
- If qualitative data is used, provide a brief summary of the themes which emerged from analysing it. Using some direct quotes from those who responded to a questionnaire or who were interviewed in the summary helps to highlight key points in the analysis and strengthens its validity.

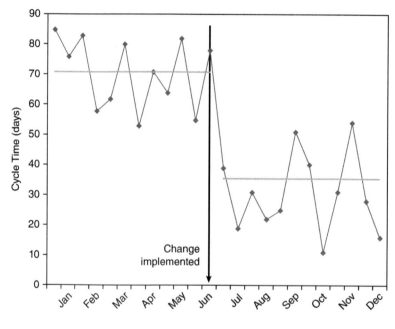

Figure 7.6   Number of days between GP referral and appointment with specialist

Source: After NHSI, 2007c, pp. 15–16.

Activity 7.8   Critical thinking and reflection

In Activity 7.4 we asked you to write down some of the issues where you work that you would like to see changed/improved. Look back now at what you wrote and identify one of these that would be appropriate for you, as a nursing associate, to lead on as a service improvement project. This might mean breaking down the issue further and focusing on one element of it. For example: you might have included some of the issues you identified in Activity 7.3 relating to waste and inefficiency that could be avoided. While some of the things you identified may be outside your own scope of practice, others may be within them. In this activity, we want you to only focus on the things that you can change.

In doing this activity, remember the Sicily Statement (Dawes et al., 2005) that we introduced you to earlier, which states that all we do should be evidence-based.

Choose one of the three models above that you could use as a framework to create your own service improvement plan. Try to justify to yourself your choice of model.

By completing the previous activities in this chapter, you will already have practised putting together a compelling case, completed a force field analysis and identified important contextual factors. Now do these activities again, but in relation to your own service improvement idea that you have identified here.

Finally, identify what baseline data you would need and the questions you would need to ask to collect them.

As this is based on your own practice, there is no outline answer at the end of this chapter.

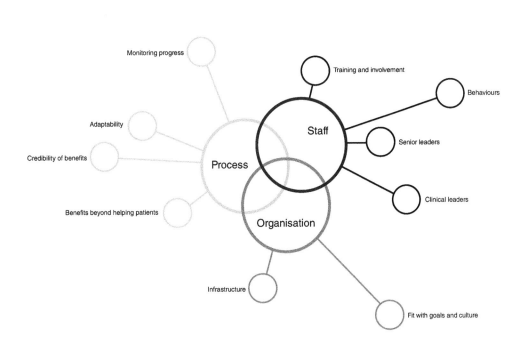

Figure 7.7   NHSI *Sustainability Model and Guide* (NHSI, 2010). See Sustainability section overleaf for more information.

Sustainability

Once it has been shown that the changes implemented do indeed represent an improvement on what was the case before, the next challenge is to maintain the improvement. Sustainability is about making sure the improvement gains stick and building upon them for further future service improvement. It is what Kotter describes as *instituting the change* to suppress any inclination to slip back to the way things used to be.

Sustaining change requires effort; it has its foundations in the way the improvement project was delivered and communicated, but just as importantly in the actions of sponsors and change leaders after the project has delivered it benefits. The NHS sustainability model (Figure 7.7) identifies ten factors which impact upon the sustainability of quality improvement projects.

Chapter summary

Dealing with change is part and parcel of working in healthcare; however, rather than it be regarded simply as something inflicted upon those working to deliver services it should be seen as a shared responsibility. Everyone involved in healthcare provision, in whatever role, including yourself as a nursing associate, should be invested in identifying opportunities for service improvement and supporting changes that lead to better outcomes for patients and service users, improved systems performance and the continued professional development that will ensure practice reflects the current evidence-base.

In this chapter we have tried to encourage you to think about what we mean by quality, the improvement of which is commonly cited in calls for change at the point of care delivery. We have introduced some key aspects of the process through which change is delivered and outlined three commonly encountered change models which can be applied within any practice environment. We have attempted to highlight the significance of the contextual influences on the implementation of change, as well as the importance of measurement in demonstrating that the changes implemented really do bring about improvement. We have also signposted you to factors which can influence the sustainability of introduced changes.

Service improvement is an essential part of ensuring evidence-based practice and is a continual process that ensures the care you and your organisation provide is contemporary – that you are not, for example, still wearing uniforms with long sleeves that you roll up but hide from matron; or wearing a belt with a buckle, as in the example of Margaret, our nurse from the 1950s. If you have successfully worked through all the activities we included in this chapter, you should now feel confident not only in being an active participant in service improvement initiatives within your own organisation, but also to lead on your own. Remember, you are the future of evidence-based healthcare delivery and can be an agent of change to ensure that it continues to be of the highest quality!

Activities: Brief outline answers

Activity 7.2 Critical thinking and reflection

Here are some things we identified, although you may have identified other/different examples. Safe:

- infection control practices such as the effective use of personal protective equipment (PPE) to reduce the incidence of MRSA and clostridium difficile (C. diff) infections;

- introduction of patient safety huddles to address issues such as falls prevention, hospital-acquired pressure ulcers and, in mental health situations, self-harm and seclusion;
- early recognition and management of the deterioration of a patient using NEWS and PEWS protocols.

Effective:

- care and treatments offered reflect current best practice in the circumstances;
- immunisation of young people against:
  - o human papillomavirus (HPV), which offers protection against HPV-related cancers, notably cervical cancer
  - o meningitis B, a common cause of infection in young children in the UK.

Patient/client experience:

- being well informed about what is happening to them;
- being involved in decision-making and care planning;
- having beliefs and wishes acknowledged and respected;
- dignity is protected; protection of modesty.

Activity 7.3 Critical thinking

Here are some things we identified, although you may have identified other/different examples. Waste/inefficiency:

- cancelled procedures due to lack of beds;
- poor communication leading to delays in provision of community services or misdirection of where they are required;
- delayed discharges due to poor organisation, e.g. required resources unavailable/delayed, such as mobility aids, take-home medication, transport, essential equipment (e.g. nebuliser);
- wasted staff time due to duplicating activities caused by poor communication or documentation, inefficient standalone IT systems, different and protracted log-in processes;
- incompatible equipment in different departments leading to waste.

Activity 7.5 Critical thinking

Examples you may have thought of here could have focused on the comfort for the nurse of not having to wear a buckle, as well as the risk of injury to the patient from the buckle.

Activity 7.7 Critical thinking

Contextual factors

Contextual factors are characteristics of a particular environment or group which combine to create something unique, despite any other obvious similarities, e.g. the type of ward.

Contextual factors can be categorised in a number of ways; Grol and Wensing (2004) use social, organisational and economic and political as sub-headings.

Social:

- the culture of the organisation, department or ward;
- the style and effectiveness of leadership;
- the values and beliefs of co-workers;
- the degree of team cohesion/collaboration.

Organisational:

- management structures, hierarchy and policies;
- effectiveness of communication systems;
- organisation and efficiency of care processes;
- multidisciplinary collaboration;
- staffing establishment, capability and skill mix.

Economic and political:

- financial arrangements;
- regulation;
- government priorities/policy.

Annotated further reading

Ellis, P (2023) Managing change, the Lewin model 1: Unfreezing. *Wounds UK*, 19(2): 69–71.

Part of a mini-series, this short article discusses the first part of Lewin's model on change management and provides a useful additional text to the material we provide in this chapter.

Metcalfe, G and Owen, A (2023) Can multiple sclerosis nurses help reduce non-elective admissions? Revisiting the question 2 years on from an analysis of a service delivery audit. *British Journal of Neuroscience Nursing (Multiple Sclerosis Supplement)*, 19(Suppl. 4): S12–S16.

This article provides an interesting read of a simple service improvement initiative that resulted in reduced hospital admissions.

Murdoch, J, Hauck, Y, Aydon, L, Sharp, M and Zimmer, M (2021) When can I hold my baby? An audit of time to first cuddle for preterm babies (<32 weeks) pre introduction and post introduction of a Family Integrated Care model. *Journal of Clinical Nursing*, 30: 3481–3492.

This is an example of a service improvement initiative and provides another interesting read of a simple service improvement initiative.

Useful websites

www.england.nhs.uk/improvement-hub/wp-content/uploads/sites/44/2011/06/service_improvement_guide_2014.pdf

This link will take you to a web-based document on improving services within the NHS. It includes the change models we describe in this chapter and will help you build on the knowledge you gain here.

https://intopractice.nice.org.uk/practical-steps-improving-quality-of-care-services-using-nice-guidance/index.html

This link will also help you build on what you have learnt in this chapter and further your knowledge, with helpful practical tips for implementing change.

www.england.nhs.uk/ourwork/part-rel/nqb/

An overview of the work of the NQB.

References

Acheson, D (1998) *Independent Inquiry into Inequalities in Health Report.* London: DHSC.

Adlam, J, Gill, I, Glackin, SN, Kelly, BD, Scanlon, C and Mac Suibhne, S (2013) Perspectives on Ervin Goffman's 'asylums' fifty years on. *Medical Health Care and Philosophy*, 16(3): 605–613.

Age UK (2023) Factsheet 62 Deprivation of Liberty Safeguards. Available at: www.ageuk.org.uk/globalassets/age-uk/documents/factsheets/fs62_deprivation_of_liberty_safeguards_fcs.pdf (accessed November 2023).

Airedale National Health Service Trust v Bland [1993] AC 789.

Avery, G (2017) *Law and Ethics in Nursing and Healthcare: An Introduction.* London: Sage.

Ball, J, Maben, J, Murrells, T, Day, T and Griffiths, P (2014) *12-hour Shifts: Prevalence, Views and Impact.* National Nursing Research Unit, King's College London.

Bates, J (2023) Hats off: Smart scrubs are a long-overdue, welcome change. *Nursing Standard*, 38(5): 12.

Beauchamp, T and Childress, J (2001) *Principles of Biomedical Ethics.* Oxford: Oxford University Press.

Beer, M and Nohria, N (2000) Cracking the code of change. *Harvard Business Review*, May–June: 133–141. Available at: https://hbr.org/2000/05/cracking-the-code-of-change (accessed June 2022).

Bibbins-Domingo, K and Helman, A (2017) Improving representation in clinical trials and research: Building research equity for women and underrepresented groups. National Academies of Sciences, Engineering, and Medicine; Policy and Global Affairs; Committee on Women in Science, Engineering, and Medicine; Committee on Improving the Representation of Women and Underrepresented Minorities in Clinical Trials and Research, Washington DC.

Bickler, PE, Feiner, JR and Severinghaus, JW (2005) Effects of skin pigmentation on pulse oximeter accuracy at low saturation. *Anesthesiology*, 102(4): 715–719.

Bolam v Friern Hospital Management Committee [1957] 1 WLR 582.

Bradshaw, P and Bradshaw, G (2004) *Health Policy for Health Care Professionals.* London: Sage.

British Thoracic Society (BTS) (2017) Guidelines for oxygen use in adults in healthcare and emergency settings. British Thoracic Society Emergency Oxygen Guideline Development Group. *Thorax: An International Journal of Respiratory Medicine*, 72(Suppl. 1): i1–i90.

Burch, J (2017) Complications of stomas: Their aetiology and management. *British Journal of Community Nursing*, 22(8): 8380–8383.

Burnes, B (2004) Kurt Lewin and the planned approach to change: A re-appraisal. *Journal of Management Studies*, 41(6): 977–1002 (accessed June 2022).

Cambridge Dictionary (2023) Cambridge University Press. Available at: https://dictionary.cambridge.org/ (accessed January 2023).

References

Care Quality Commission (CQC) (2022) CQC Medicines: Information for adult social care services. Available at: *Administering Medicines Covertly*, oacp.org.uk (accessed October 2023).

Cave, T, Ingram, D and Stein, R (2010) Improving the success rate of NHS IT projects. British Computer Society. Available at: www.bcs.org/articles-opinion-and-research/improving-the-success-rate-of-nhs-it-projects (accessed July 2022).

Chae, S, Yeo, J, Hwang, J and Kang, H (2021) Effects of school-based 'We Fit' weight control programme in adolescents. *Nursing Open*, 9: 721–732.

Charmaz, K and Thornberg, R (2021) The pursuit of quality in grounded theory. *Qualitative Research in Psychology*, 18(3): 305–327.

Child, J (2015) *Organization: Contemporary Principles and Practice* (2nd edition). Oxford: John Wiley & Sons.

Coles, E, Anderson, J, Maxwell, M, Harris, FM, Gray, NM, Milner, G and MacGillivray, S (2020) The influence of contextual factors on healthcare quality improvement initiatives: A realist review. *Systematic Reviews*, 9: 94.

Cooney, A (2010) Choosing between Glaser and Strauss: An example. *Nurse Researcher*, 17(4): 18–28.

Coughlin, M, and Cronin, P (2021) *Doing a Literature Review in Nursing, Health and Social Care* (3rd edition). London: Sage.

Coughlan, M, Cronin, P and Ryan, F (2007) Step-by-step guide to critiquing research. Part 1: quantitative research. *British Journal of Nursing*, 16(11): 658–663.

Criado Perez, C (2019) *Invisible Women*. London: Penguin, Random House.

Cummings, S, Bridgeman, T and Brown, KG (2015) Unfreezing change as three steps: Rethinking Kurt Lewin's legacy for change management. *Human Relations*, 69(1): 33–60.

Dawes, M, Summerskill, W, Glasziou, P, Cartabellotta, A, Martin, J, Hopayian, K, Porzsolt, F, Burls, A, Osborne, J and Second International Conference of Evidence-Based Health Care Teachers and Developers (2005) Sicily Statement on evidence-based practice. *BMC Medical Education*, 5(1): 1–7.

Department of Health (DoH) (2008) *High Quality Care For All: NHS Next Stage Review Final Report*. London: HMSO. CM 7432. Available at: https://assets.publishing.service.gov.uk/government/uploads/system/uploads/attachment_data/file/228836/7432.pdf (accessed April 2022).

DoH (2015) *Pressure Ulcers: Applying All Our Health Guidance*. Available at: www.gov.uk/government/publications/pressure-ulcers-applying-all-our-health (accessed January 2023).

Department of Health and Social Care (DHSC) (2021) *Liberty Protection Safeguards*. Available at: www.gov.uk/government/publications/liberty-protection-safeguards-factsheets (accessed January 2023).

DHSC (2022) Health and Care Act.

Desta, EA, Gebrie, MH and Dachew, BA (2015) Nurse uniform wearing practices and associated factors among nurses working in Northwest Ethiopia: A cross-sectional institution based study. *BMC Nursing*, 14: 1–65.

Dolan, J. (1983) *Nursing in Society* (15th edition). Philadelphia: WB Saunders.

Donoghue v Stevenson [1932] AC 562.

Eftekhari, H (2022) Ethics are central to nursing care. *British Journal of Cardiac Nursing*, 17(6): 1–2.

Ellis, P (2022) *Understanding Research for Nursing Students* (5th edition). London: Sage.

Emanuel, V, Day, K, Diegnan, L and Pryce-Millar, M (2011) Developing evidence-based practice amongst students. *Nursing Times*, 107(49/50): 21–23.

Equality and Human Rights Commission (EHRC) (2010) Equality Act 2010, c.15. Available at: www.legislation.gov.uk/ukpga/2010/15/pdfs/ukpga_20100015_e (accessed 14 December 2023); reviewed 2018.

Evidence-Based Medicine Working Group (1992) Evidence-based medicine: A new approach to teaching the practice of medicine. *Journal of the American Medical Association*, 268(17): 2420–2425.

Fitzpatrick SJ, Lamb, H, Stewart, E, Gulliver, A, Morse, AR, Giugni, M and Banfield, M (2023) Co-ideation and co-design in co-creation research: Reflections from the 'co-creating safe spaces' project. *Health Expectations*, 26 May: 1738–1745.

Francis-Devine, B (2023) *Poverty in the UK: Statistics*. House of Commons Library, UK Parliament.

Folta SC, Anyanwu, O, Pustz, J, Oslund, J, Penkert, LP and Wilson, N (2022) Food choice with economic scarcity and time abundance: A qualitative study. *Health Education and Behavior*, 49(1): 150–158.

Foster, M (2015) A guide to searching PubMed (and other free databases) for health facilities. *Design Research*, 9(1): 99–106.

Francis, R (2013) *Report of the Mid Staffordshire NHS Foundation Trust Public Inquiry*. February. London: HMSO. Available at: https://assets.publishing.service.gov.uk/government/uploads/system/uploads/attachment_data/file/279124/0947.pdf (accessed 29 November 2023).

GATE (2023) *Reaffirming Autonomy of Trans and Gender Diverse Children and Adolescents*. Available at: https://gate.ngo/wp-content/uploads/2023/07/Reaffirming-autonomy-of-TGD-Children-and-Adolescents.pdf (accessed 29 November 2023).

Goodyear, M, Krleza-Jeric, K and Lemmens, T (2007) The Declaration of Helskinki. *British Medical Journal*, September: 621–623.

gov.uk (2010) *Equality Act*. Available at: www.gov.uk/guidance/equality-act-2010-guidance (accessed 29 November 2023).

Gray, R and Sanders, C (2020) A reflection on the impact of Covid-19 on primary care in the United Kingdom. *Journal of Interprofessional Care*, 34(5): 672–678.

Gray, T (2020) Safety huddle in a community setting. *British Journal of Community Nursing*, 25(9): 446–450.

Greater Manchester Health and Social Care Partnership (2018) Greater Manchester Quality Improvement Framework. Available at: www.england.nhs.uk/north-west/wp-content/uploads/sites/48/2019/03/Quality-Improvement-Framework.pdf (accessed April 2022).

Greenhalgh, T (2019) *How to Read a Paper: The Basics of Evidence-Based Medicine and Healthcare* (6th edition). Oxford: John Wiley & Sons.

Grol, R and Wensing, M (2004) What drives change? Barriers and incentives for achieving evidence-based practice. *Medical Journal of Australia*, 180(6): 557–560.

Guyatt, GH (1991) Evidence-based medicine. *ACP Journal Club*, 114: A–16.

Guyatt, G, Cairns, J, Churchill, D, Cook, D and Haynes, B (1992) Evidence-based medicine: A new approach to teaching the practice of medicine. *Journal of American Medicine Association*, 4(17): 2420–2425.

Halliwell, C and Nayda, R (2011) Nurses' uniforms: The missing link in breaking the chain of hospital acquired infection? *Healthcare Infection*, 16(1): 24–28.

Harris, E (2022) *The Oliver McGowan Mandatory Training*, MENCAP. Available at: www.mencap.org.uk/blog/oliver-mcgowan-mandatory-training (accessed 29 November 2023).

Harris, S (2002) Japanese biomedical experimentation during World War II Era, in Beam, T (Ed.), *Textbook of Military Medical Volume 2*, Section 4: Medical Ethics in the Military. Maryland: Office of the Surgeon General.

Health and Safety Executive (HSE) (1992) *Manual Handling Operations Regulations*.

Hoffman, T, Bennett, S and Del Mar, C (2017) *Evidence Based Practice Across the Health Professions* (3rd edition). Chatswood, Australia: Elsevier.

Holland, K and Roberts, R (2013) *Nursing: Decision Making Skills for Practice*. Oxford: Oxford University Press.

Houweling, L (2004) Image, function, and style. *American Journal of Nursing*, 104(4): 40–48.

James, G (2020) *Report of the Independent Inquiry into the Issues raised by Patterson*. London: DHSC.

Jimmerson, J, Wright P, Cowan PA, King-Jones T, Beverly CJ and Curran, G (2021) Bedside shift report: Nurses opinions based on their experiences. *Nursing Open*, 8: 1393–1405.

Jones, B, Kwong, E and Warburton, W (2021) *Quality Improvement Made Simple: What Everyone Should Know About Health Care Quality Improvement* (3rd edition). Health Foundation. Available at: www.health.org.uk/sites/default/files/QualityImprovementMadeSimple.pdf (accessed April 2022).

Kapadia, D, Zhang, J, Salway, S, Nazroo, J, Booth, A, Villarroel-Williams, N, Bécares, L and Esmail, A (2022) *Ethnic Inequalities in Healthcare: A Rapid Evidence Review*. NHS Race and Health Observatory. Available at: www.nhsrho.org/research/ethnic-inequalities-in-healthcare-a-rapid-evidence-review-3/ (accessed 29 November 2023).

Kim, JH, Lim, JM and Kim, EM (2021) Patient handover educational programme based on situational learning theory for student nurses in clinical practice. *International Journal of Nursing Practice*, 24: 1–9.

Kotter, JP (2012) *Leading Change*. Boston, MA: Harvard Business Review Press.

Langley, GJ, Moen, RD, Nolan, KM, Nolan, TW, Norman, CL and Provost, LP (2009) *The Improvement Guide: A Practical Approach to Enhancing Organizational Performance*. San Francisco: Jossey-Bass.

Larson K, Jung, S and Albon, S (2019) Searching the literature: A simple step-wise process for evidence-based medicine. *Journal of Pharmacy Technology*, 35(5): 225–229.

Laurent, C (2019) *Rituals and Myths in Nursing: A Social History*. Barnsley: Pen and Sword History.

Lloyd, J (2020) Florence Nightingale: A reflection on a nurse ahead of her time. *Australian Nursing and Midwifery Journal*, 26(10): 26.

Mahmood, T (2018) What models of change can be used to implement change in post graduate medical education? *Advance Medical Education Practice*, 19(9): 175–178.

Matheson, J, Patterson, J and Neilson, L (2020) *Tackling Causes and Consequences of Health Inequalities: A Practical Guide* (1st edition). London: CRC Press.

Matthew, DB (2015) *Just Medicine: A Cure for Racial Inequality in American Health Care.* New York: New York University Press.

McBeth, C, Durbin-Johnson, B and Siegel, E (2017) Interprofessional huddle: One children's hospital's approach to improving patient flow. *Paediatric Nursing*, 43(2): 71–77.

McCormack, B and McCance, T (2010) *Person-Centred Nursing: Theory and Practice.* Oxford: John Wiley & Sons.

McGeoch, L, Ewbank, L, Dun-Campbell, K, Burale, H, O'Brien, S, Mulrenan, C and Briggs, A (2023) Briefing: Addressing the leading risk factors for ill health – framework for local government action. *The Health Foundation.* October.

McLaughlin, A (2020) *Investigating the Most Convincing Conspiracy Theories.* King's College London. Available at: www.kcl.ac.uk/investigating-the-most-convincing-covid-19-conspiracy-theories (accessed 29 November 2023).

Mencap (2007) *Death by Indifference.* London: Mencap. Available at: www.mencap.org.uk/sites/default/files/2016-07/DBIreport.pdf (accessed 29 November 2023).

Mencap (2012) *Death by Indifference: 74 Deaths and Counting. A Progress Report 5 Years On.* London: Mencap. Available at: www.mencap.org.uk/sites/default/files/2016-08/Death%20by%20Indifference%20-%2074%20deaths%20and%20counting.pdf (accessed 29 November 2023).

Mental Capacity Act (2005) London: HMSO.

Mental Capacity (amendment) Act (2019) London: HMSO.

Mikovits, J (2022) I don't feel like I'm a person: Nursing knowledge of transgender care through the lens of transgender people. *Journal of Advanced Nursing*, 78: 3012–3024.

Moen, R and Norman, C (2009) Evolution of the PDCA Cycle. Paper based on Moen, R and Norman, C (2009) The history of the PDCA Cycle. In *Proceedings of the 7th ANQ Congress,* Tokyo. Available at: https://rauterberg.employee.id.tue.nl/lecturenotes/DG000%20DRP-R/references/Moen-Norman-2009.pdf (accessed June 2022).

Montgomery v Lanarkshire Health Board [2015] UKSC 11.

Moule, P, Aveyard, H and Goodman, M (2017) *Nursing Research, an Introduction* (3rd edition). London: Sage.

Mukwende, M, Tamony, P and Turner, M (2020) *Mind the Gap: A Handbook of Clinical Signs in Black and Brown Skin.* London: St George's University.

Nairn, S, Chambers, D, Thompson, S, McGarry, J and Chambers, K (2012) Reflexivity and habitus: Opportunities and constraints on transformative nursing. *Nursing Philosophy*, 13: 189–201.

National Health Service (NHS) (2020) Uniforms and workwear guidance for NHS employers: good practice. Available at: www.england.nhs.uk/coronavirus/documents/uniforms-and-workwear-guidance-for-nhs-employers/#good-practice (accessed 29 November 2023).

NHS Digital (2023) *Reasonable Adjustment Flag.* Available at: https://digital.nhs.uk/data-and-information/keeping-data-safe-and-benefitting-the-public/gdpr/gdpr-register/reasonable-adjustments-flag (accessed 30 November 2023).

References

NHS England (2015) *The Shape of Caring Review (Raising the Bar)*. Available at: www.hee.nhs. uk/our-work/shape-caring-review (accessed 30 November 2023).

NHS England (2018) *The Learning Disability Improvement Standards for NHS Trusts*. Available at: www.england.nhs.uk/learning-disabilities/about/resources/the-learning-disability-improvement-standards-for-nhs-trusts/ (accessed 30 November 2023).

NHS England (2019) *The Long Term Plan*. Available at: www.longtermplan.nhs.uk/publication/ nhs-long-term-plan/ (accessed 11 December 2023).

NHS England (2022) *Universal Principles for Advance Care Planning*. Available at: www. england.nhs.uk/wp-content/uploads/2022/03/universal-principles-for-advance-care-planning. pdf (accessed 30 November 2023).

NHS England (2023a) *The NHS Long Term Plan. Overview and Summary*. Available at: https:// longtermplan.nhs.uk/online-version/overview-and-summary/ (accessed 30 November 2023).

NHS England (2023b) *Blue or Grey Skin or Lips (Cyanosis)*. Available at: www.nhs.uk/conditions/ blue-skin-or-lips-cyanosis/ (accessed 30 November 2023).

National Institute for Health and Care Excellence (NICE) (2015) *Pressure Ulcers, Quality Standard* [QS89]. Available at: www.nice.org.uk/guidance/qs89 (accessed 30 November 2023).

NICE (2018) *Decision Making and Mental Capacity*. Available at: www.nice.org.uk/guidance/ ng108 [accessed July 2023]

NICE (n.d.) *Involving Patients, Carers and the Public*. Available at: www.nihr.ac.uk/researchers/ i-need-help-designing-my-research/designing-research.htm#three_(accessed 30 November 2023).

NHS Institute for Innovation and Improvement (NHSI) (2007a) *Improvement Leaders' Guide: Sustainability*. Available at: www.england.nhs.uk/improvement-hub/wp-content/uploads/ sites/44/2017/11/ILG-1.7-Sustainability-and-its-Relationship-with-Spread-and-Adoption.pdf (accessed 20 June 2022).

NHSI (2007b) *Improvement Leaders' Guide: Improvement Knowledge and Skills*. Available at: www.england.nhs.uk/improvement-hub/wp-content/uploads/sites/44/2017/11/ILG-1.1-Improvement-Knowledge-and-Skills.pdf (accessed 20 June 2022).

NHSI (2007c) *Improvement Leaders' Guide: Measurement for Improvement*. Available at: www. england.nhs.uk/improvement-hub/wp-content/uploads/sites/44/2017/11/ILG-2.1-Measuring-for-Improvement.pdf (accessed 20 June 2022).

NHSI (2010) *Sustainability Model and Guide*. Available at: www.england.nhs.uk/improvement-hub/wp-content/uploads/sites/44/2017/11/NHS-Sustainability-Model-2010.pdf (accessed August 2022).

National Quality Board (NQB) (2021) *Shared Commitment to Quality*. Available at: www. england.nhs.uk/wp-content/uploads/2021/04/nqb-refreshed-shared-commitment-to-quality. pdf (accessed April 2022).

Nursing and Midwifery Council (NMC) (2018a) *The Code: Professional Standards of Practice and Behaviour for Nurses, Midwives and Nursing Associates*. Available at: www.nmc.org.uk/ globalassets/sitedocuments/nmc-publications/nmc-code.pdf (accessed 30 November 2023).

NMC (2018b) *Standards of Proficiency for Nursing Associates*. Available at: www.nmc.org.uk/ globalassets/sitedocuments/education-standards/nursing-associates-proficiency-standards. pdf (accessed 30 November 2023).

NMC (2018c) *Future Nurse: Standards of Proficiency for Registered Nurses*. Available at: www. nmc.org.uk/globalassets/sitedocuments/education-standards/future-nurse-proficiencies.pdf (accessed 30 November 2023).

NMC (2020a) *Caring with Confidence: The Code in Action*. Available at: www.nmc.org.uk/news/news-and-updates/code-in-action/ (accessed 30 November 2023).

NMC (2020b) *Professional Indemnity Arrangement*. Available at: www.nmc.org.uk/registration/joining-the-register/professional-indemnity-arrangement/ (accessed 30 November 2023).

NMC (2022) *What is Fitness to Practise?* Available at: www.nmc.org.uk/concerns-nurses-midwives/what-is-fitness-to-practise/ (accessed 30 November 2023).

NMC (2023) *We Regulate Nursing Associates*. Available at: www.nmc.org.uk/about-us/our-role/who-we-regulate/nursing-associates/ (accessed 30 November 2023).

Ong, CK and Forbes, D (2005) Embracing Cicely Saunders's concept of total pain. *BMJ Clinical Research*, 331(7516): 576.

Øvretveit, J (2009) *Does Improving Quality Save Money? A Review of the Evidence of Which Improvements to Quality Reduce Costs to Health Service Providers*. Health Foundation. Available at: https://health.org.uk/sites/default/files/DoesImprovingQualitySaveMoney_Evidence.pdf (accessed June 2022).

Øvretveit, J. (2011) Understanding the conditions for improvement: Research to discover which context influences affect improvement success. *BMJ Quality and Safety*, 20 (Suppl. 1): 18–23.

Øvretveit, J, Andreen-Sachs, M, Carlsson, J, Gustafsson, H, Hansson, J, Keller, C, Lofgren, S, Mazzocato, P, Tolf, S and Brommels, M (2012) Implementing organisation and management innovations in Swedish healthcare: Lessons from a comparison of 12 cases. *Journal of Health Organisation and Management*, 26(2): 237–257.

Owens, M (2015) An exploration of collaborative practice and non-formal interprofessional education by medical and nursing students in the primary care setting. Doctorate of Education thesis, University of Huddersfield.

Parahoo, K (1999) A comparison of pre-Project 2000 and Project 2000 nurses' perceptions of their research training, research needs and of their use of research in clinical areas. *Journal of Advanced Nursing*, 29: 237–245.

Park, L (2020) Using the SBAR handover tool. *British Journal of Nursing*, 29(14): 812–813.

Parker, T and Carlisle, C (1996) Project 2000 students' perceptions of their training. *Journal of Advanced Nursing*, 24: 771–778.

Pechy, R and Monsivais, P (2016) Socioeconomic inequalities in the healthiness of food choices: Exploring the contributions of food expenditures. *Preventative Medicine*, 88: 203–209.

Peters, MDJ, Marnie, C, Tricco, AC, Pollock, D, Munn, Z, Alexander, L, McInerney, P, Godfrey, CM and Khalil, H (2020) Updated methodological guidance for the conduct of scoping reviews. *JBI Evidence Synthesis*, 18(10): 2119–2126.

Piano, MR (2017) Alcohol's effects on the cardiovascular system. *Alcohol Research*, 38(2): 219–241.

Pistella, J, Ioverno, S, Rodgers, M and Russell, S (2020) The contribution of school safety to weight-related health behaviours for transgender youth. *Journal of Adolescence*, 78: 33–42.

Power, A (2015) Ensuring practice is based on the best evidence: A masterclass on literature searching. *British Journal of Midwifery*, 23(5): 356–358.

References

Public Health England (PHE) (2018a) *Research and Analysis. Chapter 5. Inequalities in health.* Available at: www.gov.uk/government/publications/health-profile-for-england-2018/chapter-5-inequalities-in-health (accessed 30 November 2023).

PHE (2018b) *Density of Fast Food Outlets.* Available at: www.gov.uk/government/publications/fast-food-outlets-density-by-local-authority-in-england (accessed 30 November 2023).

Pun, J (2021) Factors associated with nurses' perceptions, their communication skills and the quality of clinical handover in the Hong Kong context. *BMC Nursing*, 20(95): 1–8.

Rao, TS and Andrade, C (2011) The MMR vaccine and autism: Sensation, retraction, and fraud. *Indian Journal of Psychiatry*, 53(22): 95–96.

Redfern, M (2001) *The Royal Liverpool Children's Inquiry Report.* London: HMSO. Available at: https://borninbradford.nhs.uk/what-we-do/cohort-studies/bib-family-cohort/_(accessed 30 November 2023).

Royal College of Nursing (RCN) (2017a) *Essential Practice for Infection Prevention and Control.* London: RCN.

RCN (2017b) *Accountability and Delegation.* Available at: www.rcn.org.uk/professional-development/accountability-and-delegation (accessed May 2023).

Ryan, F, Coughlan, M and Cronin, P (2007) Step-by-step guide to critiquing research. Part 2: qualitative research. *British Journal of Nursing*, 16(12): 738–744.

Sackett, DL, Rosenberg, WM, Gray, JA, Haynes, RB, and Richardson, WS (1996) Evidence based medicine: What it is and what it isn't. *British Medical Journal*, 312: 71.

Seedhouse, D (2017) *Thoughtful Healthcare: Ethical Awareness and Reflective Practice.* London: Sage.

Shbaklo, N, Lupia, T, De Rosa, FG and Corcione, S (2021) Infection control in the era of Covid-19: A narrative review. *Antibiotics* (Basel), 10(10): 1244.

Shuval, K, Linn, S, Brezis, M, Shadmi, E, Green, ML and Reis, S (2010) Association between primary care physicians' evidence-based medicine knowledge and quality of care. *International Journal for Quality in Health Care*, 22(1): 16–23.

Sjoding, MW, Dickson, RP, Iwashyna, TJ, Gay, SE and Valley, TS (2020) Racial bias in pulse oximetry measurement. *New England Journal of Medicine*, 383: 2477–2478.

Soofi, H (2022) Respect for autonomy and dementia care in nursing homes: Revising Beauchamp and Childress's account of autonomous decision-making. *Bioethical Inquiry*, 19: 467–479.

Spragley, F and Francis, K (2006) Nursing uniforms: Professional symbol or outdated relic? *Nursing Management*, October: 55–58.

Stimpfel, AW, Sloane, DM and Aiken, LH (2012) The longer the shifts for hospital nurses, the higher the levels of burnout and patient dissatisfaction. *Health Affairs (Project Hope)*, 31(11): 2501–2509.

Tanner, R (2022) *Unfreeze, Change, Refreeze: Is This a Child's Game?* Available at: https://managementisajourney.com/unfreeze-change-refreeze-is-this-a-childs-game/ (accessed August 2022).

Taylor, SL, Dy, S, Foy, R, Hempel, S, McDonald, KM, Øvretveit, J, Pronovost, PJ, Rubenstein, LV, Wachter, RM and Shekelle, PG (2011) What context features might be important determinants of the effectiveness of patient safety practice interventions? *BMJ Quality and Safety*, 20(7): 611–617.

Thomas, J (1985) Force field analysis: A new way to evaluate your strategy. *Long Range Planning*, 18(6): 54–59.

Thompson, C, Cullum, N, McCaughan, D, Sheldon, T and Raynor, P (2004) Nurses, information use, and clinical decision-making: The real worlds potential for evidence-based decisions in nursing. *Evidence-Based Nursing*, 7(3).

Tobin, M (2022) Fiftieth anniversary of uncovering the Tuskegee Syphilis Study: The story and timeless lessons. *American Journal of Respiratory and Critical Care Medicine*, 205(10): 1145–1158.

UK Research and Innovation (2021) Talking about Covid conspiracy. *Sense about Science*. Available at: https://senseaboutscience.org/activities/talking-about-conspiracies/ (accessed 30 November 2023).

Valbuena, V, Seelye, S, Sjoding, M, Valley, T, Dickson, R, Gay, S, Claar, D, Prescott, H and Iwashyna, T (2022) Racial bias and reproducibility in pulse oximetry among medical and surgical inpatients in general care in the Veterans Health Administration 2013–19: Multicenter, retrospective cohort study. *British Medical Journal*, 378: e069775.

Vosoughi, S, Roy, D and Aral, S (2018) The spread of true and false news online. *Science*, 359(380): 1146–1151.

Wade, C, Malhotra, AM, McGuire, P, Vincent, C and Fowler, A (2022) Action on patient safety can reduce health inequalities. *British Medical Journal*, 376: e067090.

Watson, A (2017) Lewin's change management model vs Kotter's 8-step model. Together Abroad. Available at: www.togetherabroad.nl/blogs/3/qee4wt-lewin-s-change-management-model-vs-kotter-s-8-step-model (accessed 10 August 2022).

Wensing, M, Grol, R and Grimshaw, JM (2020) *Improving Patient Care: The Implementation of Change in Health Care*. Oxford: Wiley-Blackwell.

West, S (2019) Blog: Role differences between nursing associates and nurses. Available at: www.nmc.org.uk/news/news-and-updates/blog-whats-a-nursing-associate/ (accessed 30 November 2023).

Williams, E, Buck, D, Babalola, G and Maguire, D (2022) *What are Health Inequalities?* London: Kings Fund.

World Health Organization (WHO) (n.d.) *Social Determinants of Health*. Available at: www.who.int/health-topics/social-determinants-of-health#tab=tab_1 (accessed 30 November 2023).

WHO (2022) *Global Competency Framework for Universal Health Coverage*. Available at: www.who.int/publications/i/item/9789240034686 (accessed 30 November 2023).

Wounds UK (2021) *Best Practice Statement: Addressing Skin Tone Bias in Wound Care: Assessing Signs and Symptoms in People with Dark Skin Tones*. Available at: https://wounds-uk.com/wp-content/uploads/sites/2/2023/02/191ac9b79f47de2896cf1a30f39037f5.pdf (accessed 29 November 2023).

Index

NOTE: Page numbers followed by "f" indicate figures; those followed by "t" indicate tables.

Abdoli, S, 40
accessibility of information, 76, 79–80
Accident and Emergency departments, 60
advance decision to refuse treatment (ADRT), 89
Advanced Care Planning (ACP), 89
advertisements, 53, 59
age assessment, 89
Airedale National Health Service Trust v Bland, 87
Allied and Complementary Medicine Databases (AHMED), 21
anthropology, 41
appropriate person, 89
autism, 20, 32, 76, 80
autonomy, 93

Babalola, G, 73
Beauchamp, T, 93
Bécares, L, 75
believability, 56, 61
beneficence, 93–94
best interests, 96
    assessment, 89
    care plan, 87–90
Bibbins-Domingo, K, 78
Bolam Test, 87
Bolam v Friern Barnet Hospital Management Committee, 87
Boolean operator, 22, 23, 23t
Born in Bradford (BiB), 36, 37, 46
Bosom, M, 38
British Journal of Nursing, 27
Brown, D, 54
Buck, D, 73

capacity, consent, 87
Care Quality Commission (CQC), 92
case control study, 37, 49
case studies
    care, 12–13
    ICU/HDU force field analysis, 107, 108f
    Jim, 84–85
    Margaret, 9–11
    Simon, 18–19, 25–26
    Toni, 32–33, 35, 44
Chae, S, 52, 57, 58, 62–68
Change as Three Steps (CATS), 106–108
Charmaz, K, 42

Childress, J, 93
CINAHL database, 21
clinical expertise, 7
clinical negligence, 86–87, 96
Cochrane, A, 8
cognitive behavioural therapy (CBT), 36
cohort study, 36, 46–47, 48
consent to treatment, 87–90, 96
conspiracy theory, 20
contextual awareness, 112–113
contextual factors, 102, 117–118
coordinated approach, 103
COPD, 79, 81
Coughlan, M, 56, 58, 61t
Court of Protection, 89
COVID-19 pandemic, 20, 75, 78, 104
Crenshaw, K, 76
Critical Appraisal Skills Programme (CASP), 56, 57
critiquing research, 55–59
Cronin, P, 56, 58, 61t
crossover randomised control trial, 36

database searching
    adding structure to, 23–25
    reliable evidence, finding, 20–23
decision-making, 84
    consent, mental capacity and best interests, 87–90, 96
    duty of care and clinical negligence, 86–87, 96
    ethical, 92–94
    ethical dilemmas, 94–95
    legal accountability, 86
    professional accountability, 85–86
Declaration of Helsinki, 43
deductive approach, 34–35
Deming, WE, 110
demonstrable improvement, 113–115
deprivation of liberty (DoL), 88
Deprivation of Liberty Safeguards (DoLS), 88, 89
discrimination, 74–76
    racism, 76–77
    sexism, 10, 76–77
diversity in healthcare, 72
doctor, as source of evidence, 19, 20, 28
Donoghue v Stevenson, 86
double-blinded randomised control trial, 36
drivers of change, 104–105
duty of care, 86–87, 96

eligibility assessment, 89
Ellis, P, 52, 57–58
Equality Act (2010), 72, 73, 74, 77
ethical considerations, 43–44, 56
ethical decision-making, 92–93
    autonomy, 93
    beneficence, 93–94
    justice, 94
    non-maleficence, 93
ethical dilemmas, 94–95
ethnography, 41, 49
evidence
    in contemporary practice, 17–30
    database searching, 20–23
    reliable, finding, 20–23
    sources of, 19–20, 26–28
    triangulating, 26, 28
evidence-based healthcare, 1, 6, 9, 10, 11, 100, 105, 116
evidence-based medicine, 8–9
evidence-based person-centred care, 1
evidence-based practice (EBP), 1, 6–7
    1850s, Nightingale, Florence era, 8
    1970s, Cochrane, Archie era, 8
    1990s, Guyatt, Sackett and Project 2000, 8–9
    defined, 7–8
    health inequalities and, 72–73, 75–76
    historical development of, 8–11
    at present, 9–11
    and research, 19
    timeline for evolution of, 7f
    traditions, routines and rituals, 11–13
    See also decision-making
evidence-informed practice, 9
experimental study. See randomised control trial (RCT)

Fitzpatrick, K, 41
force field analysis, 107, 108f
Francis Inquiry, 12

Galantino, G, 38
Goffman, E, 41, 43
Goldacre, B, 55, 62
Google Scholar, 21
Granger, K, 80
Grol, R, 117–118
grounded theory research, 42, 48–49
Guyatt, G, 8–9

handovers, 10–11, 14
Health and Care Act (DHSC), 76, 80
health inequalities
    defined, 73–74
    and evidenced-based practice, 72–73, 75–76
healthcare support workers (HCSW), 6, 11, 13
Helman, A, 78
high-level drivers, 104
high-quality personalised care, elements of, 102, 116–117
Hwang, J, 52, 57, 58, 62–68

ICU/HDU force field analysis, 107, 108f
impact factor, 27, 28

inductive approach, 38–39
informed consent, 87
Institute for Healthcare Improvement (IHI), 110
integrated care systems (ICS), 104
intersectionality, 76–77
Ioverno, S, 35, 37, 38, 46, 56

Jim case study, 84–85
journal article, as source of evidence, 19, 27
justice, 94

Kang, H, 52, 57, 58, 62–68
Kapadia, D, 75
King, ML, 72
Kotter's eight-step change model, 109–110, 116

The Lancet, 20
Langley, GJ, 110
lasting power of attorney (LPA), 89
learning disability, 76, 80
legal accountability, 86
Letby, Lucy case, 20
Lewin's change model, 106–108
liberty protection safeguard (LPS), 84, 89, 90
life expectancy, 73, 75

Maguire, D, 73
Margaret case study, 9–11, 14
Matthew, DB, 75
McCance, T, 91
McCormack, B, 91
McGlashan, H, 41
McGown, O, 76
Medico, D, 38
MEDLINE database, 21
Mencap, 76
mental capacity, 96
    assessment, 89
    and best interests, 87–90
    Mental Capacity (Amendment) Act 2019, 90
    Mental Capacity Act 2005, 88, 92
mental health assessment, 89
Mid Staffordshire NHS Trust, 12, 13, 80
Mikovits, J, 52, 57, 58, 62–68
Model for Improvement, 110–112, 111f
Moen, RD, 110
Montgomery v Lanarkshire Health Board, 88
Mukwende, M, 81
multidisciplinary team (MDT), 14, 19, 90, 91–92, 100

National Health Service (NHS), 74
    NHS Choices, 19, 28
    NHS England, 61, 75, 76, 101, 104
    NHS Health Research Authority, 43
    NHS Institute for Innovation and Improvement (NHSI), 103, 110, 115f
National Institute for Health and Care Excellence (NICE), 26, 94
National Institute for Health Research (NIHR), 44
National Nursing Research Unit, 14
National Quality Board (NQB), 101, 112
neighbour principle, 86

newspaper, as source of evidence, 19, 20, 26–27
Nightingale, F, 8
no refusals assessment, 89
Nolan, KM, 110
Nolan, TW, 110
non-experimental study. *See* cohort study
non-maleficence, 93
Norman, CL, 110
North American principles, 43
Numerical Rating Scale, 36
Nursing and Midwifery Council (NMC), 12, 85
 Future Nurse: Standards of Proficiency for
  Registered Nurses, 9
 NMC Code, 6, 6f, 18, 32, 85–86, 87, 90,
  92, 101
 revalidation and practice development, 73
 Standards of Proficiency for Nursing Associates,
  1, 2–3, 9, 84, 85–86, 87, 92, 101

Oliver McGown Training, 76
open access, 55
organisational change, steps for, 109–110
Øvretveit, J, 103, 112

patient
 experience, 101
 involvement in research, 44
 safety, 101
 as source of evidence, 19, 27
 values, 7, 11
Patterson, Ian case, 20
PCC tool, 23, 24t, 25, 28, 29–30
Perez, CC, 78
person-centred care
 evidence-based, 1
 working in partnership with others, 90–91
phenomenology, 40, 48
PICO tool, 23, 24t, 25
PICO(s) tool, 23, 24t, 25, 28–29
Pistella, J, 35, 37, 38, 46, 56
Plan-Do-Study-Act (PDSA) model. *See* Model
 for Improvement
primary data, 19
primary research, 19, 32
probability, 54
professional accountability, 85–86
Project 2000, 8–9, 11
Provost, LP, 110
PsycINFO, 21
publication bias, 55
PubMed, 21, 22
pulse oximetry, 78–79, 81

qualitative research, 37–38, 38f, 57–58, 68
 checklist for, 61t
 ethnography, 41, 49
 grounded theory research, 42, 48–49
 inductive, 38–39
 other types of, 42
 phenomenology, 40, 48
 subjectivity and objectivity, 39–40
 terminology, 39t

quality
 defined, 101
 key elements of, 101
 nature of, 101–103
 single shared view of, 102, 102f
 See also quality improvement
quality improvement, 100
 changing, 105–106
 contextual awareness, 112–113
 defined, 103
 demonstrable, 113–115
 drivers of change, 104–105
 equation, 103–116, 104f
 evidence-based, 105
 Kotter, John steps for leading organisational
  change, 109–110
 Lewin's change model, 106–108
 Model for Improvement, 110–112, 111f
 quality and, 101
 sustainability, 116
quantitative research, 35f, 57–58, 68
 case control study, 37, 49
 checklist for, 61t
 cohort study, 36, 46–47, 48
 deductive, 34–35
 other types of, 37
 randomised control trial, 35–36, 48
 terminology, 39t

racism, 75, 76, 81
randomised control trial (RCT), 35–36, 48, 60
reasonable care, 86, 87
registered nursing associate, 85–86
research
 critical thinking about, 52–55
 critiquing, 55–59
 ethics, 43–44
 evidence, 7, 8, 55, 78, 90, 92, 94, 95
 robustness, 58, 61
 sense of, 32–33
 service user (patient) involvement in, 44
 See also qualitative research; quantitative research
Roach, A, 40
Rodgers, M, 35, 37, 38, 46, 56
Russell, S, 35, 37, 38, 46, 56
Ryan, F, 56, 58, 61t

Sackett, D, 9
Sansfaçon, A, 38
scientific method of enquiry, 110
secondary data, 19
seminal pieces, 22
sex discrimination, 10
sexism, 76–77
Shape of Caring Review (NHS England), 75
Sicily Statement, 105
Simon case study, 18–19, 25–26
situation, background, assessment and
 recommendation (SBAR), 11, 14
social determinants of health, 74–75
social gradient, 75
social media, 20, 27

Index

Soofi, H, 94
specialist website, as source of evidence, 19, 27
stereotypes, 77
subjectivity and objectivity, 39–40
Suerich-Gulick, F, 38
supervisory body, 88, 90
sustainability, 116
sustainable use of resources, 103
systematic approach, 103, 105

therapeutic intervention, 35–36
Thomas, S, 40
Thornberg, R, 42
Toni case study, 32–33, 35, 44
transgender, 32–33, 35, 41, 46, 52, 68
transparency, 55
truncation, 23
Trust/organisation policies, as source of evidence, 19, 28
Tuskegee Syphilis Study, US, 43

unconscious bias, 77, 78–79
Unfreeze – Change – Refreeze. *See* Change as Three
    Steps (CATS)

uniforms, nursing, 10, 14
utilitarianism, 94

Visual Analogue Scale, 36
voluntary consent, 87

Wakefield, 20–21
Wensing, M, 117–118
Wikipedia, as source of evidence, 19, 28
Williams, E, 73
working in partnership with others
    multidisciplinary team, 91–92
    person-centred care, 90–91
World Health Organization (WHO), 26, 72, 73
    Competency Framework, 9
    social determinants of health, defined, 75
Wright, M, 40

Yates, A, 40
Yeo, J, 52, 57, 58, 62–68
YouTube, 53, 54, 55, 57, 62, 91

Zufferey, A, 38